I0476704

Have Medic,
Will travel.

By: Spike Bowan

Disclaimer: these stories are true! All names, dates and places have been changed to protect the privacy of individuals involved and no privacy laws are violated.

This book contains graphic content and situations and is not intended for young eyes!

Be a good parent and don't let your little ones read this until they are much older.

If you do, you are dumb and a prime example of Darwinism at its finest.

This book is intended for entertainment/ educational purposes. It is an insight to what emergency crews actually do and go through. If that is too hard to swallow, or you're offended, too bad. This is what happens in the real world. Come out of your ivory tower and wake up!

Special thanks to:

My wife and my son, you are my soul, my inspiration and my reason for continuing to be the one running towards the screams. I live and fight, for you.

CHRISTMAS COMPRESSIONS:

December 24th,

    I had just become an EMT in October. The ambulance service I joined was very short on volunteers for the holiday, and being sixteen with no life besides the fire hall and video games, I jumped at the chance to run emergency calls over the holiday. The weather outside is cold and dreary. Snow is falling, but not really sticking to the roads. The day didn't provide many calls for the two full Paramedic crews that were stuck with the holiday shift. The crews and I sit around the dining table enjoying a ham that was brought in by one of the board members. We discuss topics from local sports, to what we want for Christmas.

    I jump like there is no tomorrow! The pager and alarms scare the crap out of me!

    "EMS respond, to the apartments on Main Street for an elderly female patient, not responsive, not breathing"

    The crews jump up, including myself, and scramble towards the ambulances. The garage doors open, the trucks start up. The rumbling of the diesel engines vibrates my soul. My heart is beating one hundred miles an hour as the emergency lights turn on and the sirens blare. The trucks pull out of the garage and head down Main Street. Weaving in and out of holiday traffic. Narrow misses with people that seem to forget to pull their cars over for the ambulance, get my heart beating faster.

    As we arrive on scene, the Paramedic on my truck tells me to grab the "Jump Bag" and the Cardiac monitor. "Damn thing weighs a ton!" I say to myself. The five of us scramble into the apartment building. This place was not designed with the thought of ambulance crews getting a patient in and out of here on a stretcher. The elevators can only fit three of us. Don't even think about getting a stretcher in here. It wouldn't fit if your life depended on it, and this old lady's life just might. We have to send the first group up and then send the lift back down for the rest. I am on the first ride up. The door opens on the floor we need and as we exit, I can see the narrow hallway is filled with people. We politely make our way down to the apartment. Apologizing, and excusing ourselves for the equipment bouncing off the people in the hallway.

The apartment is tiny. Barely enough room to live let alone have a family get together for the holiday. Sons and daughters, Grandkids, nieces, nephews, brothers and sisters, the apartment is packed full of family. The smell of holiday cookies and eggnog fill my nose as the sounds of the families' cries and sobs fill my ears. A man directs us toward the bedroom. "She said she wasn't feeling good and went to lay down" the man says. "I went to check on her a few minutes later and that's when I noticed my Mother stopped breathing" he states.

I enter the bedroom behind my Medic. She reaches down and feels the patient's carotid artery for a pulse. "Nothing." She said. "Move her on to the backboard and begin compressions" she tells me. Really, Oh my God! Umm I have never done CPR before. I do as she says. The patient is tiny, I am only sixteen, but even I can lift this eighty-pound woman to the floor by myself. I place the patient on the board with help from the other EMT. I find my hand placement, I breathe. ***CRACK*** my first compression almost makes me cry. The feeling of the cartilage in her chest breaking under my hands is unlike anything I have ever felt before. It felt like breaking pasta to put in a boiling pot of water. A sensation I have never fully gotten used to in twenty years.

The other crewmembers arrive after about a hundred years of me doing compressions on this patient. In actuality it's only been two minutes, but it feels like a lifetime. My Paramedic gets her equipment together to intubate the patient. The other Paramedic starts an IV as the EMT's prepare to extricate the patient on a Reeves stretcher. The reeves is a collapsible canvas stretcher that is more pliable and maneuverable around the tight corners. The crews work, I compress on the chest. I hear family crying, screaming at us to do something, anything! One family member screams, "THEY'RE KILLING HER!" "Killing her? Fuck you man! She was already dead and we're trying to save her!" I say in my head.

The chaos that is a cardiac arrest is always one of high emotions and tempers. "Patient is in V-FIB (Ventricular Fibrillation), I'm gonna shock her!" my Medic exclaims with authority. She grabs the paddles of the defibrillator, charges them, and places them on the chest of the patient as I stop compressions. The thought of that much electricity surging through the body scares me.

"CLEAR!" ***THUNK*** "CHARGING, CLEAR!"***THUNK*** "CHARGING 360! CLEAR!"***THUNK*** "ASYSTOLE, CONTINUE COMPRESSIONS!"

The smell of the charged flesh in my nose makes my stomach turn. I place my hands again and compress. Again and again and again I push on this ladies chest. Trying to get even the tiniest response back from her heart. The Medics are pushing drugs left and right. Epinephrine, Atropine, Sodium Bicarbonate.

They have intubated the patient and are giving medications and oxygen down the tube and through the IV catheter. I keep compressing. My arms feel like mush. I have been doing these chest compressions forever, I say to myself. It's actually only been a few minutes. One of the EMT's relieves me on the patient's chest and tells me to go get the elevator and hold it open.

As I stand up, I feel the tingling of pins and needles in my hands. I shake them to try and regain feeling. I excuse myself past an onslaught of onlookers. All family, the looks I get are a barrage of emotion. Fears, pain, anguish, contempt, hatred, hope, confusion, so many looks thrown my way all at the same time. I try to shrug them off as I head toward the elevator down the narrow hall.

A button push and a few minutes of me standing there holding the door later, here comes the two crews. Doing CPR and ventilating the patient as they move. We cram the patient, one medic and myself in the elevator. The rest of the crews head down the four flights of stairs to meet us at the bottom. I take over compressions, straddling the patient in the cramped elevator. Occasional cracks and pops still occur as I compress the patients' chest. The feel of this is still making me cringe. The elevator is taking forever because we stop on every floor on the way down. Apparently the whole damn building needed to use the elevator at the same time. Imagine their surprise as the doors open and they see a Paramedic and a green EMT performing CPR on a patient. One guy on the second floor even said "Merry Christmas". "Really? Wow!" I say as I look at the Medic. She chuckles and tells me, "You'll see some weird shit in EMS kid!"

We finally arrive at the bottom floor where the rest of our brethren are waiting with the stretcher. We transfer the patient and resume CPR. By this time we have a third Paramedic on scene who operates a Quick Response Unit out of the local hospital. He takes my place, as the patient is loaded into the ambulance. The QRS Medic looks at me and says, "Hey kid! You have a license?" "What...uh. Yea...yes." I fumble over my own words as he throws me the keys to his Emergency unit. "Don't wreck it kid." I pause in pure confusion as I look at the keys in my hand, turn and see an old Ford Bronco with Emergency Lights. This is a big sport utility vehicle! "I drive a Chevette for heaven's sake! You want me to drive that beast?" I exclaim in terror. "Like I said, don't wreck it kid!" He closes the door as his words ring in my ear. No pressure. No pressure at all. Who am I kidding, my hands are still shaking at the feeling of that woman's chest crumbling under them, and now I am driving a tank.

The ambulance drives off leaving the Sherman Tank and me on scene. I move toward the two-ton behemoth. The snow is falling down heavier now and starting to cover the road. Of course it is. I have to drive General Patton's personal chariot! I enter the driver side door and start up the monster of a vehicle. Seatbelt, check. Mirrors check. Scared to fucking death, check. Let's do this. I put her into gear and begin to drive toward the hospital, which is four miles away. Wow, this is pretty easy and the cars on the road are getting out of my way. On a narrow street too. I wonder...HOLY SHIT THE EMERGENCY LIGHTS ARE ON! I panic and fumble, trying to find the off switch and not wreck the Paramedic Panzer! I am not doing so well at the light finding objective and decide to just go with it. Now, I am building a little confidence and I feel it. I feel like a Bad Ass! I look good and I am driving the USS Missouri down Main Street!

I pull into the Emergency room parking lot and park the truck. As cool as I can, I strut into the emergency room. Cocky and with a swagger in my step, I stroll in. I did CPR today. I drove a Tank. I am awesome! The arrogance of a sixteen year old is quickly crushed when I see the ER staff scrambling to save this woman, the EMS crews tired and out of breath, and the family. The family looking at me, the crews, the ER staff, crying and praying for a miracle. It's Christmas Eve, and their mother, sister, grandmother, aunt and friend is dead. I fall to my knees right next to the room. The sheer fact that I could be so self-absorbed while this family lost one of their own is appalling. I pray, right there and then. "God let your will be done. Forgive my sins and arrogance, ease the pain of this family and let them make it through this holiday knowing that she is in a better place. Amen."

I rise to my feet as the Doctor exits the room, pulling off his exam gloves he shakes his head. The nurses do the same. I peer into the room and see the little old lady lying there. Empty and hollow, one last nurse pulls a sheet over the head of the body. A tear rolls down my cheek as I turn to see the doctor and a priest talking to the family. It is this moment, that I swear to God and myself that I will be a Paramedic. I will help the families out there to the best of my ability. No longer will I act so foolishly. I will put others before myself.

My heart heavy, I walk outside and light a cigarette. A few moments pass and the snow is coating almost everything. The streetlights are reflecting off the fresh and fluffy snow. I think about all that has transpired and am feeling a little lost. I hear footsteps crunching in the snow when a voice calls to me, "Hey kid, you have another cigarette?" I grab one from my pack and hand it to, the son. Damn, the son of the lady who just died and had originally directed us into the room.

I hand him the cigarette and offer him a light. Not knowing what to say, I am silent. "Thanks kid." He says. I nod and try not to make eye contact. After a couple of drags off his smoke, he looks at me and says, "How old are you kid" and me, I look at him now replying, "16" "16, are you kidding me?" I am waiting for him to go on a tangent. A rant about how some snot nosed kid is trying to play superhero with his mothers' life. These words never leave his mouth, instead he says, "Wow kid. 16 and you're here on Christmas Eve trying to save my mother's life. You're not at home with your family or girlfriend; you're out in the cold, doing CPR on my mother. I wish there were more kids like you in the world. You never gave up on her; you and your crewmembers went above and beyond kid. Thanks for the Christmas present." He turns, throws out the cigarette, and leaves.

I don't know what happened, but I can only think of one thing. This is what I am supposed to do for the rest of my life.

The first time I did CPR, it was Christmas Eve, a lady died, I drove a Tank, God quickly corrected me in my arrogance and I got the best Christmas present I could have ever had asked for at that time.

The Train and the VETERAN:

One night in early summer, I was finishing up a shift and it is close to midnight. The off going crews are standing around the garage next to the ambulances talking to the oncoming crews and enjoying the evening air with the garage doors open. I am at the far end of the garage talking to the off going medic from the response vehicle that the local hospital stations at our base. Nice guy. He knows his stuff and he has an amazing bedside manner. We talk about my leaving next week to go to Advanced Individual Training (A.I.T.) for the U.S. ARMY Reserves next week. I will be gone for 10 weeks in Alabama. I had finished my Basic Training (BOOT CAMP) Last summer and then returned to graduate from High School. I am not too thrilled about going, because I wanted Combat Medic and it wasn't available so I got Ammunition Specialist with the hope of transferring once Medic opened up again. My partner, who is also my Fire Chief at the Volunteer Company I run with, stands at the other end of the garage. A large and jovial guy, his laugh is unmistakable. Chief is a standup guy though. Always teaching me what is what and looking out for me. I was very happy to be teamed up with him for the shift.

As we stand there and talk, I see a man walking a dog down the road and he heads directly towards the Response Medic and myself. The guy looks ragged. His hair is unkempt and he has no shirt on. Only a military flight jacket that is covered in unit and campaign patches. His cut-off denim shorts are stained, filthy and they don't hide the scars on his legs. His feet are housed in dilapidated work boots that have more holes in them than laces. He approaches walking his yellow lab, the dog is on a rope instead of a leash. About six feet away I notice that he has a 1st Calvary patch on the shoulder of his flight jacket and Vietnam service patches, as well as a Combat Infantry Badge. In my head I think, "DAMN! This guy saw some shit!" I quickly dismiss my thought as the man starts to tie the rope leash off to the downspout of the building. He speaks.

"Do you guys know the animal shelter in the next town over?" he says this shaking. "Yea man, what about it?" I say being very confused. "Can you make sure my dog gets there? He is a good boy and very friendly. His name is Huey." The veteran starts to back up away from us. "What's going on sir? How come you can't keep him?" as I say this the veteran starts to back up further, "Because I am going to kill myself!" He runs in a panic. I look at the Response Medic and he looks at me, and as clear and unmistakable the train horn blow. ***HONK*** our eyes get huge as I scream for my partner who is at the other end of the garage still.

"CHIEF!" I scream at the top of my lungs, much as a Drill Sergeant would at the new recruits. My partner turns and looks, "That guy is going for the train!" I bellow as I jump into the response unit with the Medic. Emergency lights on, we fly out of the garage and pull out into the street blocking off traffic. The train tracks run parallel to the station across a busy roadway. Past the train tracks is the lock and dam on the river. The Veteran heads down the hillside and stands on the tracks. "This is bad!" The Medic says as he grabs the radio to let dispatch know what is going on. I exit the vehicle and stand on the embankment next to the tracks. Calling out to the Veteran, my voice is drowned out by the blare of the massive diesel train that is barreling down toward the Veteran. He can't hear me. I move down the hill. Closer to him, and the train.

By this time all that is going through my head is that this guy is not dying tonight. I will not let this happen. "What's your name bud?" I try to confidently ask him. Inside I am shaking, trying to think of how to reach this guy. He doesn't reply. His eyes are fixated on the massive iron horse charging towards him. It isn't even slowing down. A voice in my head screams, "Veteran, play the Veteran card!" "At Ease Soldier!" I shout. The Veteran turns to me in surprise and retorts, "What do you know about the military, you are just a kid!" "Kid, not so much, I am a Private 1st class in the Army Reserve. I also come from a long line of veterans." A brief pause and the Veteran steps off the tracks toward me. I step back a few paces trying to keep a safe distance. As much as I want to help this guy, I don't want to end up under the train either. "You joined?" he says in disbelief. I nod. "You don't know what it is to be a Combat Veteran! You haven't seen the shit I have!" "You are right. I haven't, yet. My time will come soon enough, and I have many family members that have seen what you have. I know how bad it can be. Talk to me sir. Let me help you." I plead with the man to talk.

His gaze is now up the hill at the 4 ambulances and six police cars. There was even a State Trooper present. They all stay up on the hill. Ready to rush in and help if need be, however they let me talk to the Veteran.

"I don't want to go to jail. I just want it to be over. It hurts, so badly. The dreams, the head aches, I try to explain it to people. And the... sound blares, and then the smoke...because you have to do a check before you fly...and then mosquito's get in and the smoke chokes you...you sweat and sweat and sweat, when you wipe it away it's red... everyone is screaming...WHY IS EVERYONE ALWAYS SCREAMING AT ME!" He shouts at me in a synaptic break that sends his body to its knees shaking, crying.

His eyes puffed out and full of tears he looks up at me. Clearly this man, this Soldier, this Veteran has never received the help he so desperately needs. With a tiny voice, and his hands lying in one another he says to me, "I pray that you never have to be in my shoes son. No one listens to the homeless guy who has nightmares." I lower to one knee; "I am here. I am listening."

For the next thirty minutes, we sit and talk. Life, the service, his injuries, I let him vent. The police try to make their way down to us a couple of times and I wave them off. This Veteran is hurting. He is not a drug addict, or a psychopath. He is a man that has seen and experienced things that a person should never have to. The thought that we, as a people could ignore and disregard someone who fought for our country and allows him or her to end up in this position disgusts me.

"The hospital down the road has people that will listen to you too." I state. "I'm not going to jail?" he asks still sobbing. "No brother, you are not going to jail." He stands up with help from me, "Alright, I will go with you." Hand in hand we walk up the hill toward the platoon of emergency responders that await us.

I lead him to the ambulance and let him have a seat on the stretcher. One of the oncoming crewmembers pulls me aside. "You are a fucking Idiot!" He screams at me. "That guy could have grabbed you, thrown you under the train, shot you or stabbed you! You're a dumb ass!" He keeps screaming at me and pushing his finger into my chest. "I didn't see you down there! Where were you, oh yea, cowering behind the line of police you fucking coward! I was not letting this man die tonight! So Fuck You!" I push right back with all the conviction in my being, knowing I did the right thing. As Mr. Douche Bag tries to puff up his chest at me, my partner steps in between us. "It's all good, he was speaking military with the guy and there is no bloody mess to clean up. All is good. And you were hiding behind the cops dude!" my partner says as he motions me to the truck to go sit in the back with the Veteran. I told you my Chief was a stand up kind of guy.

A short ride and brief conversation later, we arrive at the hospital and I transfer care of my new friend to the hospitals psychiatric staff. The police took the dog to the animal shelter. He was a nice dog too. I never saw the veteran or the dog again. Never heard anything else about him either.

I was left with a feeling of humility and sorrow. And fear. Fear that the mental state of this decorated Veteran, could be me someday. The next week, I was on a plane to Alabama to complete my job training for the U.S. Army.

ICE CREAM:

I have been running for several months with my new ambulance company. Located in one of the busiest urban suburbs. They average anywhere from 7,000 to 10,000 calls a year. Shootings, stabbings, domestic assaults, drug overdoses as well as a lot of head scratching medical calls. This station is just about the same pace as when I was a Corpsman in the Navy. Busy, very busy with barely the time to eat let alone complete paperwork. I love it here! The staff is elite; there isn't a single person in the employ of this rescue company that I wouldn't trust with my life or my family's lives.

It's a mid-summer day and the sun is shining in the sky, mixed with the heat that is bouncing off the blacktop to meet in the middle creating a sweat filled uniform. Yes, definitely like the Navy. My partner, I and the rest of the crews have been steady all day. On a humid day like today we get our fair share of respiratory calls. Asthma and Chronic Obstructive Pulmonary Disease (COPD) don't like humidity. The other city crew just returned from a call, so we're next up. I try to get paperwork and reports organized as the minutes pass. The crews are trying to relax while there is some down time. We try to enjoy what little of these breaks we get by watching the news, smoking a cigarette and talking about sports. The usual water cooler behavior applies.

"Damn it!" I exclaim out loud. The pager and station bells ring.

***MEDICS RESPOND TO FRANKLIN AVENUE FOR AN UNKNOWN AGE CHILD, STRUCK BY A VEHICLE! ***

I am immediately up and out the door grabbing my radio and stethoscope as I run to the truck. Pediatric calls always get my adrenaline pumping. More so now that I have a child of my own. It's hard not to look at an injured child and not think about my son. On the way to these calls I have to breathe and remind myself that he is safe and at home.

The lights of the ambulance shine their eerie red shadow on the wall of the garage as the door opens. The diesel engine rumbles alive and my partner pulls the truck out of the station calling enroute to the 911 dispatcher, "Medic 6 enroute to Franklin". The siren plays our theme song of high and low tones as we race down the road. As per usual people seem to forget to yield to an emergency vehicle as we have to serpentine through traffic. The buildings and house's whiz by, a blur of abandoned homes and run down porches fill my peripheral vision. We make the bend on to the main road passing the hospital and try to avoid hitting a telephone pole that has at least four pairs of sneakers hanging from its wires. We almost hit it because some schmuck wouldn't pull over.

"Pull to the right DUMB ASS!" my partner screams out the opened window. The dispatcher calls and gives us an update.

MEDIC 6, BE ADVISED, POLICE ON SCENE STATE THAT THE CHILD IS APPROXIMATLEY 6 YEARS OLD AND IS LOSING CONSCIOUSNESS WITH SHALLOW RESPERATIONS

I already suspect a number of injuries that can cause this in the child. I grab the radio and call the dispatcher back. "Dispatch, Medic 6 copies, get a chopper on standby" It's a child, he sounds bad, it's rush hour and we are thirty minutes away from the children's hospital in normal traffic. Damn right I want a helicopter! We head busily down the road. I can feel my heartbeat in my throat. As we approach the scene I see a cadre of police cars and a geriatric assistance bus with a child lying in front of it. "Oh, God! A bus hit him"

That's precisely what happened. I scramble out of the rig as I apply my gloves and head toward the child my partner grabs the cervical collar and backboard. He's barely conscious and his brief moments of lucidity are spent crying in a low murmur. "Hey buddy, open your eyes. C'mon kid open your eyes!" I try to rouse him. He manages to open his eyes part way and there it is. His left pupil is fully dilated and his right pupil is pinpoint. I call on the radio to have the chopper meet us at the landing zone. The compression in the child's skull is severe and located right in the middle of his occiput (back of the head). Cerebral spinal fluid is leaking from his ears. This is bad.

The story I get from the police as I work on the child with my partner and a second EMS crew that has now arrived on scene is as follows.

The child's mother was sleeping, and the child couldn't wake her when he wanted some ice cream. "Probably because of the crack cocaine she had just smoked as indicated by paraphernalia found in the residence" the officer states. So the child took money out of her purse and decided to walk down the road to a convenience store to get his ice cream. Franklin is a very busy street. People speed down it all the time. The child apparently walked right out in front of the bus. The driver had no time to react, and he wasn't even speeding. Speed limit and a big bus equal a recipe for disaster to a 6-year-old boy.

I frantically try to stabilize this boy. We have the child immobilized on the backboard with a cervical collar. His pelvis appears unstable and I think he might have a femur fracture. As we load the child into the back of the ambulance, one of the other EMT's already has my supplies out to start an IV (Intravenous catheter). The Paramedic from the second truck hops up to take the airway seat and starts giving the child oxygen. I prepare my supplies and apply a tourniquet. Surprisingly, the child has remarkable veins for a 6-year-old boy. My needle slides into his skin with the greatest of ease. He doesn't even flinch. I start administering fluids through his IV, which is now secure. Another crewmember put the electrodes on his chest and I glance at the screen of the monitor.

The peaks and valleys of green waveforms move so fast that they can cause your eyes to blur. His little heart is beating so fast. "Sinus Tachycardia on the monitor" I state to the Paramedic at the head of the patient, who is squeezing the bag valve mask. "End tidal CO2 is 37"he replies. Children are resilient creatures. Their bodies can compensate for damage and illness for a long time before it crashes. This kid is no exception. His blood pressure is low; we're replacing fluids. His respiration's are fast, we're helping control them with the bag mask and pure oxygen. His ETCO2 (end tidal carbon dioxide) levels are stable, which means his lungs are function properly by blowing of acid. If we can stabilize the rest of him, his heart rate will hopefully normalize. His head is a different story. Dollars to Pesos, I'm betting he has a skull fracture.

The ambulance doors slam shut with a vengeance and the tires smoke as the driver, probably my partner, begins hauling ass to the landing zone. We continue to keep an eye on all of the child's vital signs and try to talk to him. "Hey bud, are you with us?" no response. Unconscious. Damn it! The trip to the landing zone is only a few minutes away, less with "Evil Kenevil" behind the wheel. My partner is in the wrong profession. This guy should be a NASCAR driver. He has crazy awesome driving skills. We tear through the streets of our fair hamlet, driving like madmen. The whole time another Paramedic an EMT and I work desperately to help this little boy.

We pull up to the landing zone. The helicopter is already on the ground. Rotors still turning, the crew of the evac chopper knows that this will be a "load and go" situation. The flight crew enters the back of the rig. We judiciously transfer the boy to their equipment as I relay a care report to the flight nurse. Their stretcher, their monitor, we help maneuver the litter to the helicopter. Hunkered down as to not get our heads cut off by the blades of the rotor, we navigate the grassy and muddy terrain with little problems. The flight crew loads the boy into the helicopter and we scurry back to our ambulance on the sidelines.

A few moments pass, and the helicopter takes off in a hurry. The down draft from the propellers is immense. Dust and debris fly about. My eye gazes upward watching them as they fly away. "Dude, our truck is trashed!" my partner says with a tone of hating the cleanup that is to follow. The other Paramedic comes up to me; my eyes still fixed on the tiny dot on the horizon that was the helicopter. "Are you alright?" he says. The two of us standing there covered in the blood of a little boy. Exhausted from the sheer crash of the adrenaline rush that has just bid me farewell.

I turn to him, coming back to my senses and the only thing I can say to him are the following eight words.

"All he wanted was a fucking ice cream."

The cricket:

It was really hot this one summer. The humidity and rising temperatures make for very unpleasant shifts. I would have to change my socks and underwear several times a shift because they would become so soaked, that to not do so was an open invitation to athletes foot and crotch rot. Our crews ragged, we have been running calls all day. Heat strokes, asthma attacks, there was little time to rest and drink water to hydrate ourselves. My partner and I are driving down the road with the air conditioner on full blast. The chill from the man-made cooling is a welcome change of pace from the inferno that lies just a few millimeters outside the truck door.

Almost back at the station, we receive a call from dispatch.

MEDIC 15 RESPOND. HURST AVENUE FOR A 40 YEAR OLD FEMALE WITH CHEST PAIN AND SHORTNESS OF BREATH

"Medic 15 copies, enroute to Hurst Ave." my partner flips the lights and turns on the siren. Hurst is only a few blocks from the station. Our arrival on scene takes little time. "Medic 15 on scene dispatch". I open the truck door being met with a face full of devil breath that is the temperature outside. I instantly miss the Chevy refrigerator I just left. Cardiac monitor and jump bag (AKA first in bag or medical bag) in hand, I progress toward the residence. Old newspapers line the porch and the mailbox hasn't been emptied in a few days. The red brick town house is in dire need of repair. Shudders, shingles and gutters all need replaced. I open the screen door as my partner approaches with the oxygen bag. ***KNOCK, KNOCK, KNOCK*** "Medics!" I call out.

I hear a muffled voice through the door that sounds distant. I knock again, banging the door and frame harder with my fist and repeat my previous phrase. Again, a muffled voice tries to reach me through the door. I reach down and turn the doorknob again opening the cheaply composed door. "Hello, Medics" "Up here!" the voice shouts to me from up the filth covered stairs. The house is a pigsty. Garbage bags filled with trash, stacks of magazines and old newspapers line the walls. The air smells of cat feces, ammonia, probably old urine from the cats or who knows what else and cigarettes. I almost vomit on the floor immediately. The smell of this house is so repulsive that part of me wants the fire department to come to let me use one of their air packs. Mix the aroma of ashtrays, animal excrement, rotting trash along with the scolding temperatures outside and I already know this call is going to suck ass.

We haphazardly make our way up the stairs to follow the sounds of this meek voice beckoning us to help. I crest the stairs to find the upstairs is worse than the downstairs. Cockroaches scurry about the walls and floors. Thousands of them, in broad daylight. Again, I almost vomit. We shimmy past the stacks of clutter in the hallway to a bedroom. Nothing on Gods amazing Earth could prepare me for what I saw next. "Please help me, I don't feel well."

Here my patient sits. Morbidly obese and filthy, puffing away on a cigarette, ashtray sitting on her enormous naked stomach. This lady weighs at least 500 pounds. The crust of what looks like the filling from a cream filled sponge cake is firmly dried itself to the area around her mouth. She is completely naked, sitting on her bed that is stained in urine, feces and possibly blood. The whale of a patient takes a long creepy drag off her smoke, taking it all the way down to the filter and extinguishes it in the receptacle sitting on her belly. I have no words. Seriously, the words can't even form in my mouth to begin the patient interview. She looks at us waiting for somebody to say something. She retrieves another cigarette from her pack and lights it up. I shake my head back to the subject in hand and am about to talk to her when I notice it. A cockroach, crawling down her forehead.

She brushes it aside and ignores the vermin with a gesture that this occurs on a regular basis. Now I know I am about to vomit. "Ma'am, you called the ambulance? What seems to be the problem today?" I am trying not to run out of this cesspool screaming right now. "I have chest pain and it's hard to breathe. Been this way for three weeks!" she drags of her cigarette to the point you would think that she needs the nicotine more than air. She probably does. "Three weeks, what changed between three weeks ago and today that you felt the need to call an ambulance?" she takes another drag off her cigarette and slowly reaches down between her legs to scratch herself. She starts to answer me as she pulls her hand back up and sniffs her fingers. My partner turns around and runs downstairs to leave me with this exemplary specimen of humanity and the reason humans are top of the food chain.

It speaks.

"Well, there is nothing on TV today, and I figured the hospital was better than watching 'Baywatch' re-runs." This woman doesn't even care that she is a putrid disgusting thing. All manners and any semblance of nice disappear from my behavior from this point on. "Ok, do you have something to put on so I can walk you downstairs to the stretcher?" I am trying to be polite. "I ain't fucking walking! You're gonna carry me down those damn steps!" I don't even miss a beat, "Like Hell I am! That isn't even remotely gonna happen! Get up, cover up for the love of God, and let's get out of your...house!" I move to the hallway and wait. After a few moments, she waddles out of the bedroom, still smoking and we start to head downstairs. The whole time she is screaming obscenities at me. "You lazy mother fucker, won't do your job and carry his patient down these God damn steps. You're done asshole, I am gonna have your job, you're gonna get fired...etc."

I should bite my tongue, but screw that! I have been standing in a hovel that would make a sewer rat vomit. "That's enough! Shut up lady! You waited for three weeks to call an ambulance for chest pain and shortness of breath. Meanwhile you're sitting in your dirty house naked and smoking a pack of cigarettes in front of us, and you're out of breath? Then you say there's nothing on TV so the hospital would be more interesting? Are you kidding me? Let's go! Stop talking, you're out of breath remember?" a bit much, I really lost all tact that I ever possessed.

She grumbles, and makes her way out the door and down the front steps of the residence. She plops her butt on the stretcher, which my partner had retrieved, from the truck. We gather the equipment and strap the patient to the stretcher. We both nearly get a hernia loading her into the truck. Her hair is matted and filled with chunks of dried food, ash from her smokes and the occasional cockroach. She reeks like a bakery. The candida yeast that forms in all of her crevices is overpowering in the back of an enclosed space. I hurry and start the IV, give her some Aspirin, which is part of the chest pain protocol. Even though she has had this "pain" for three weeks, a little aspirin won't hurt anything. I apply the electrodes of the cardiac monitor. She mumbles insults under her halitosis filled breath. Her body is filthy, absolutely disgusting. I lift her left breast with gloved hand to apply the electrodes for a twelve lead EKG.

"JESUS HELP ME, WHAT THE FUCK WAS THAT?" I scream as something flies past my head, missing my face ever so slightly. I turn to look at the wall of the ambulance behind me. Sitting there, looking at me is a cricket. Alive and well, chirping. I kick open the back door of the ambulance and proceed to vomit. "Oh, now that's real professional!" her remark pisses me off so badly I shoot her an evil look in between my heaves of vomit. Once completed, I look at my partner and tell him to get us to the closest hospital, yesterday. Lights and sirens, and approximately 1000miles per hour, we were at the hospital before you knew we left the scene of the horrid house.

I have never had such a quick turn over in the Emergency Room. I wanted to get away from that woman as fast as possible. My partner is way ahead of me, having grabbed mops, a broom and bleach. We clean the rig as fast and thoroughly as possible. Then, a scream! Followed by more screams! We run into the ER to see what happened. The sight before us is almost comical as we see a nurse and a medical student vomiting in separate garbage cans in tandem. The attending resident comes up to us, somewhat squeamishly. "What happened Doc?" I say. The resident takes a moment to compose himself. Finally he says, "We were applying electrodes for our own EKG and insects started pouring out from the folds of her skin and under her breasts!"

We look at the floor and see cockroaches and the occasional cricket hopping around. We ran out of that ER so fast, that I left my clipboard on the nurse's station. I hurry back, grab it and ran back out. We speed back to base. We have a small fistfight over who gets to shower first. I won. As the evening went by, we tell the other crewmembers the story after dinner. They don't believe us, shouting profanities about how much we're lying. We tease each other and then there is a silence at the table. A brief respite, then our guest of honor shows up for dinner.

The cricket jumps onto the dinner table.

We weren't lying guys.

THE CRASH:

On a beautiful spring evening, my partner the other crews and I were sitting down to dinner at a local restaurant. It's my last shift here and my thoughts are everywhere but work. We are all sitting around talking and joking. Waiting for our food is always a never-ending task. The food never seems to come until you light up a cigarette. Sure enough, just as I do, here comes my cheeseburger and fries. The topic of current discussion among the crews is summer vacation. Seeing as I was leaving for the Navy in two days to become a Hospital Corpsman, I wasn't involved much in the chat.

The diner wasn't overly busy, a steady flow of patrons come and go, people brush past each other, a plate breaks in the distance and some knucklehead customer starts clapping and cheering at the waitress. Berating her for the accident as if we were in high school. "What a prick!" I say aloud. The conversation among the crews comes to a halt. You know the part in a movie where someone says or does something and the background music screeches to a halt and everyone in the room looks at that person. That's what this felt like. "What? Who? Who's the prick Spike?" my partner asks me with a look of confusion. "What? Oh, that guy in the corner, the teenage 40 year old that clapped and cheered at the waitress as she broke the plate. I hate people like that. That's all." The "music" restarts and the movie continues with everyone returning to the place in their confabulations.

"So, why the switch Spike?" the question seems to be emanating from the entire table. My thought process drifts back to reality to answer the question posed. "Army reserves just ain't cutting it for me. I am gonna be a Combat Hospital Corpsman with the Marines. I made some calls, jumped through hurdles and am now doing a lateral conversion. I lose some rank, but that's ok. I guess I feel like I am supposed to go."

"You'll do fine, don't come back with a husband though, we know how those sailor boys are!" My partner's joke isn't appreciated. In fact I think his dad was a Gunners Mate on ship in Vietnam. Ironic really.

The truth is, my Grandfather just died and my girlfriend told me that I was the "other guy" and she had been cheating on her long time fiancée with me. She tells this to me on the night I was going to propose to her and the bitch left me standing there with a ¼ karat diamond ring in my pocket. She was out of my league anyway, too high maintenance. I will miss the sex though. Girl was an animal in the sack. I just felt like I would never get out of Pittsburgh, never do something with my life or achieve anything of significance, unless I did something drastic. Active duty Navy Combat Hospital Corpsman with the Marines is as about as drastic as I could come up with. My grandfather wanted me to see the world, and live. He said there was more to life than just Pittsburgh. I was gonna find out.

I come back to the world and begin eating my dinner. The boisterous asshole from the corner finishes his meal and walks past us toward the register to pay for his food. Everything about this guy screams jerk. Just one of those guys that the instant you meet him you want to break his jaw. I choose to ignore his existence and enjoy my burger. Over the next few minutes we chat and finish our meals. We take our turns at the register and pay for our food. Shuffling our feet towards the rigs, we saunter over.

The pagers wake us out of our food-induced comas.

"Medic 5, Medic 6 respond, to the Elm Street Bridge for a multiple car vehicle accident, with entrapment. Multiple injuries being reported, police and fire department are enroute."

"County Medic 5 and Medic 6 are on the way, is that the East or West end of the bridge?"

"Medic 5, Medic 6, be advised, this is in the middle of the bridge."

My partner revs the engine, I flip the switch and we are gone. A blur of sirens and lights, our trucks fly down the road. We serpentine through the traffic and red lights. A chaotic ballet of driving and near misses. We arrive at the bridge, which was only a few blocks from the diner and we can see smoke towering above one of the vehicles halfway across the bridge. The traffic is backed up on both sides, and there is no easy way to get to the scene. We park our trucks at the West End of the bridge and load up all of our equipment on the stretchers and hurry down the walkway on the bridge.

After a few feet my partner looks and sees the flames coming from one of the vehicles and that the fire engine is blocked all the way at the East End of the bridge. "Spike, go get the extinguisher from the bus!" I nod and double-time it back to the rig. I grab the extinguisher from its carrier and hustle back to the stretcher, which is almost down to the scene of the accident. As I approach, I see that it is not the accident holding up the traffic, but one guy in a pickup truck that is just sitting in the middle of the bridge blocking both lanes of traffic, and he is taking pictures.

My partner rushes to the first car and the Medic 5 crew rushes over to the second vehicle, a pickup truck. I pull the pin on the extinguisher and begin to hose down the two engine compartments that are now fused together from the impact. The fire subsides and the Medic 5 crew makes their way to our car. "He's dead." The medic states, "His head broke through the windshield. Even if that didn't kill him, his face being directly in the fire and his eyeballs exploding did."

That settles that, we now have two full crews with their attention on the driver and passenger of the remaining vehicle. We evaluate the driver as Medic 5 crew takes the passenger. The drivers head is split down the middle, almost perfectly in half by a piece of metal rebar that was in the back of the other vehicles truck bed and must have flown forward with the impact. Killing the driver of our vehicle instantly. No pulse, no brain matter left. Yea, he's dead. The Medic 5 crew and my partner focus on the passenger.

The woman has part of her scalp ripped back. She bit through her own lower lip. Multiple fractures and her legs are pinned underneath the dashboard. I can even see part of the engine block sitting on her legs. "We need rescue in here to cut and roll the dash" I say to my partner. "I agree," he says. "Make it happen" and with his words I exit the car to evaluate logistics.

"County, from Medic 6. We need heavy rescue in here to extricate the patient. We have 2 victims DOA. Have rescue expedite and have a chopper at the LZ of the football field."

"Medic 6, that's received"

I look at how I am going to get that rescue truck here and realize that pickup truck is still blocking the bridge and its driver is still taking pictures. I move toward the truck and my jaw drops. It's the asshole from the diner! "Hey! Shit Head! Get the Fuck out of here! What the hell is wrong with you?" I scream at the jerk as I motion for him to move his vehicle. He peers up from behind his camera and smiles as he says, "Fuck you!" Without a pause I run to his driver side door ripping it open. I grab his camera and throw it over the bridge into the river. "You're gonna pay for that!" he punches me in the jaw. The guy hits like a bitch. I drag him from his truck and slam him against the side. "These people are dead and she is dying, we need a rescue truck in here and you are taking pictures! Do you really think I care about your camera or the fact you hit like a bitch? Get into your 'Ass Hole Mobile', and get the fuck off my scene!" I reaffirm my rant with another slam of his back against the truck.

The Ass Hole contemplates his next move and then re-enters his truck. Shifting into gear he peels tire and speeds off. "Wow, the guy even drives like a bitch." My thought makes me chuckle. The rescue truck arrives and the firefighters begin to work their magic. My partner and the other crew are stabilizing the lady. The crunching of the metal and the smell of hydraulic fluid from the rescue tools makes for a weird and horrific memory. One I soon won't forget. Especially when we find a newborn baby, dead under the dash. The mother must have been holding the baby on her lap when the collision occurred. The engine block crushed the baby's skull and the rest of the child was so mangled that I couldn't tell which way his head was facing.

The mother died on the way to the landing zone.

Four dead. I couldn't help but wonder, if at least one of them could have lived if that ass hole from the diner had not parked in the middle of everything to get some snap shots.

THE RASH:

It had been a busy shift. My partner and I are running ragged. Call after call. We go and we assess, we fix and we transport. We had just cleared up from one call and get toned out for another.

"MEDIC 7 RESPOND, TO EDGAR TOWERS, PD ON SCENE REQUESTING MEDICS. UNKNOWN AGE FEMALE PATIENT WITH AN UNKNOWN MEDICAL PROBLEM"

"Medic 7 acknowledges and enroute." I furiously replace the radio microphone back in its holder. It is midday and already this is our sixth call since the beginning of the shift. We make our way to the high-rise known as Edgar Tower. "I wonder what's wrong with the lady. Probably a junky or an assault victim." My partner has a valid point. The tower contains some of the most miserable dregs of society. We are constantly called to this area for assaults, overdoses and the like. We also get a lot of people with serious medical conditions that are unable to take care of themselves. Diabetics that don't eat or take their insulin, CHF (congestive heart failure) and COPD (chronic obstructive pulmonary disease) patients that chain smoke three packs of cigarettes a day.

It is a short trip to the high-rise from where we were. We arrive on scene to find multiple police vehicles in front. My partner and I look at each other, "This might suck." "Medic 7 on scene with Police. Do we have a better location on the patient dispatch?" I gather my clipboard and put on a pair of exam gloves. "MEDIC 7 BE ADVISED THE PATIENT IS IN THE RENTAL OFFICE OF THE BUILDING." "Medic 7 copies", my partner grabs the jump bag, and we enter the tower.

As we enter the lobby, the smell of stale urine and cigarettes fill my nose. My olfactory senses now rattled and completely offended we climb the stairs to the next floor where the rental office resides. We enter through the office door and are directed to the rental manager's office by the secretary. Two left turns in the cramped office and we see the rental manager sitting behind her desk. "Here she is gentleman." The manager points to a chair by a bookcase where our patient is resting. "The police are here for another matter and they saw this lady and called you guys."

My first response is pure shock. I have traveled all over the world and seen many horrendous things. This is one of them. The patient, we will call her "Itchy", is in her mid to late 50's and is frail in stature. Top to bottom, front to back and side to side she is absolutely covered in a purple blotchy crusty rash. Her face is bleeding in certain areas where she has scratched the skin entirely away. She has literally peeled the skin off from her own face. She twitches and scratches at herself. Her actions are of pure discomfort and she leaves very little of herself unscratched. I can only imagine that she must feel like the lepers of old.

"Hi, how long have you had this rash?" I am trying to remain calm and not appear scared that she is a walking contagion. "A few days. I was hoping it would go away on its own and it hasn't." She scratches her arms raw in front of us. "You haven't been playing with any armadillos have you?" I try to quip with her and all I receive is confusion, from Itchy and from my partner. I then had to explain that leprosy (a.k.a. Hansen's disease) could be transmitted to humans from armadillos according to studies. It can also be transmitted from human to human via respiratory droplet exposure. She lightly chuckles at my attempt at humor "No, no armadillos. I only got my new medicine this week." If this were a cartoon, I would have a light bulb over my head right now.

"What new medicine?" I already have a sneaking suspicion I am just waiting for Itchy to give me the other piece of the puzzle. "My psych doctor changed my 'Haldol' from a pill to a long term injection."

"WINNER WINNER CHICKEN DINNER!"

Steven Johnson Syndrome (SJS) is a mild form of Toxic Epidermal Necrolysis (TEN). It is an idiopathic (not known, pertains to that specific patient) presentation where cellular death in the skin causes the epidermis and the dermis to separate. Both of these if left untreated can be deadly. Although both SJS and TEN can also be caused by infections, they are more commonly adverse effects of medications. It is not contagious that I know of and both diseases can be mistaken for erythema multiforme. Erythema multiforme is sometimes caused by a reaction to a medication, but is more often a type III hypersensitivity reaction to an infection (caused most often by Herpes simplex) and is usually benign. **(See Wikipedia and American Academy of Dermatology)**

My partner retreats to the ambulance as I explain what I think this rash may be to Itchy. Itchy stands up and gathers her things. I notice that the chair where she was sitting is covered in purple skin flakes. We make our way down to the elevator and I can't help but be infatuated with such an appalling disease process. Her skin looks like purple refried beans that sat in the refrigerator uncovered for a couple days. Except there is blood oozing out of the crusty nodules. I feel bad for Itchy. Her road to recovery from this will be long. It can take months for her skin to heal. That is if she doesn't die in the process.

We begin transport to the local emergency room, which is only a few blocks away. As we arrive at the hospital, we escort Itchy in and immediately receive disgruntled looks from one of my least favorite doctors. This guy is a world class schmuck. He looks at Itchy and instantly talks about transferring her to another hospital. He grumbles and gripes. I have never in all of my years met a doctor that hated Paramedics and Nurses so much. I think he even hates the other ER doctors. This jerk and I have gone rounds before. I am very grateful that I haven't followed through with my daily urge to kick his ass. He bullies Itchy into an exam room and rips the exam curtain to the side.

I look at my partner, he looks at me and we shrug our shoulders simultaneously. We turn and head toward the exit. We never knew what happened to Itchy, but every now and then I see Dr. Schmuck scratch his arm and I just have to laugh.

Karma dude.

Karma.

THE AMPUTATION

I have been working for this private ambulance company for over a year. The crews are filled with good people. The pay is amazing, probably for a lack of decent equipment. The bad part about this company, is the fact that not only do we have to run emergency calls in the surrounding four towns but we are contracted with dozens of private facilities around the county for their emergency calls. So if your grandmother is at an extended care facility, and she needs an ambulance, we could be coming from the other side of the county. It pays the bills.

I am in Medic 231. My partner is a good guy. We have known each other for years and are now working together here at this private company. We joke and talk about the hockey game last night as we are returning from the city after completing a transport. We notify our company's private dispatcher that we are clear of the transport and are returning to the area. We have a ton of paperwork to do and the truck still needs washed. The traffic on the parkway is as thick as molasses in winter.

We sit idle, and wait forever to move six inches. All because people in this damn city are afraid of the tunnels that lead in and out of it. "I wish people would just drive! THERE IS NO TUNNEL MONSTER THAT IS GOING TO EAT YOU! MORONS!" I get very frustrated with Pittsburgh drivers. "Calm down Spike. You're on the clock anyway." My partner's reassurance actually worked. I am getting paid good wages to sit in traffic. No it didn't, I am bored, my butt is numb and the yuppie (rich person) in the Mercedes next to my window is jamming to 'Lady Gaga'. I want to shoot someone.

"STATION 230 RESPOND. TO THE INTERSECTION OF 3RD AND MAIN STREET FOR AN UNKNOWN AGE MALE PATIENT WITH AN ARM AMPUTATION."

"Holy Shit! Are you kidding? And we are stuck in traffic. Oh well." I haven't had a messed up trauma in a while. I would have loved to get that call. "Dispatch, Medic 238 enroute" we listen as 238 calls enroute and gets on scene quickly. They must have been at the station. Within thirty seconds Medic 238 calls back in service. Angrily I might add. I look at my partner with a raised eyebrow. "What the hell was that all about?" All six of the trucks have been busy today, transports and emergency calls keep coming so I can understand 238's attitude, but thirty seconds on scene is either a really bad call or it was complete bullshit. "What do you think? Bad or Bullshit?" my question doesn't even take a minute to settle in my partners thoughts. "Bullshit." He is usually right.

What would normally be a twenty minute drive back to station takes the better part of an hour. All because of the "Tunnel Monster". As we make our way through the tunnels we finally reach our exit. That was an excruciating traffic jam. We have the rest of our brief trip to review the day, and joke about a certain nurse at the one emergency room that my partner has a crush on. She's cute. Too tall for me though. We pull into the garage and the first thing we see is Baker, one of the other Paramedics, he is screaming his head off. He is stomping around much like a 2-year-old with a temper tantrum. "Wasn't Baker on 238?" my partner nods in disbelief.

I jump out of 231 and walk towards Baker. I shout to grab his attention, "Hey Baker! What's wrong man?" "Spike, this is HORSE SHIT! That guy, that FUCKING GUY! If I see him, I will kill him. I will rip off his 'missing arm' and beat him to death with it!" Baker's words make little sense but his 'finger quotes' are funny. Baker proceeds to tell me the following story.

"We pull up at the intersection expecting to find a guy with his arm lopped off. Instead we find this guy standing there with two arms like the most of men. We walk up and the guy is holding a piece of paper. I ask him if he called the ambulance. He says 'yea man. I called you guys.' 'What happened to your arm?' 'Nothing, I just said that shit so you fuckers would get here quicker.' Then the guy lifts up the piece of paper and says, 'can you fill my prescription?' Spike, I almost beat the shit out of the guy, but instead of going to jail I told him to 'FUCK OFF CRACKHEAD!' and then we left. I can't believe these people Spike. This is HORSE SHIT!"

I had to laugh in disbelief at Baker's story. I give the crackhead points for originality, but blatant abuses of the health care system like this occur daily. When I say daily, I mean thousands and thousands of times a day. All across the United States. People will call saying they have chest pain and request to go to a hospital on the far side of town. When they get there, they sign out AMA (against medical advice) just because they needed a ride and didn't have cab fare, bus money or Jitney money. (Jitney is what an illegal cab service is called in Pittsburgh) Some people don't even go into the hospital. They will hop off of the stretcher and walk out of the hospital parking lot.

I look at Baker and look at my partner and the only thing I can say to them is "Good thing you didn't transport him Baker, that bill would have cost him an 'Arm and a leg'!"

THE COFFEE BREAK

The day was long and boring. We hadn't been all that busy and my partner laid down in the bunk room and passed out from sheer apathy. The EMT from the other crew and myself sit around and watch TV, twiddle our thumbs. Whatever passes the time. I can almost tell the time by the rhythmic snoring of my partner. Each inhalation and exhalation are perfectly synchronized and in tempo. His snoring sounds like a tank driving over an elephant. My friend, Ally is the other EMT on the other medic truck. She is a really fun girl and a damn good EMT. She and I are talking about nursing school. She has been pulling her hair out over some of the pathophysiology topics. I sit there and try to help her to the best of my ability, but some of the things a nurse is required to learn make little sense. A huge portion of the things they learn in school they will never use or need in a practical setting.

"STATION 25 RESPOND, EMERGENCY, TO MORRIS RETIREMENT APARTMENTS, FOR A MEDICAL ALARM ACTIVATION. UNKNOWN AGE MALE, COMPLAING OF CHEST PAIN, POSS HEART ATTACK. POLICE ARE ENROUTE."

The emergency call comes in when both of our partners are sleeping. Her Paramedic and my EMT are in deep sleep. So, it's either waking them and deal with having grumpy partners for the rest of the shift or take the call together and get it done. We look at each other and without saying a single word we nod and silently agree to take the call together. We grab our coats and make our way to the truck room. My "new" partner is only about five and a half feet tall and is part Libyan and absolutely gorgeous. She walks with a confidence that is hard to find in most U.S. Marines. Being that we work in one of the worst ghettos in the county, a petite angel, that can kick ass, comes in handy. She knows her medicine and can handle herself. I couldn't ask for a better partner. We saddle up and get into my rig.

"County dispatch, Medic 251 enroute to Morris Apartments."

We start to drive. It's not that far of a distance. The apartment building we need to respond to is right at the bottom of the hill from the station. Right past the hospital. It is a quaint little complex in the middle of the ghetto. A place for older people that have the ability to function on their own but can't maintain a whole house by themselves can live. We usually get the occasional fall, chest pain or diabetic emergency from here. Nothing like the three section eight housing facilities we have to cover. There, we get nothing but childbirth, drug overdoses, assaults, and gunshot wounds. Welcome to the way of the world. We quickly zoom down the hill arriving at our destination with haste.

"Dispatch, Medic 251 on scene."

A friend and police officer for our city meets us on scene. Mitt is a good cop. I would not want to be on the receiving end of this man's wrath. I tower above him both height and build wise, but he is tenacious. He has a ferocity that is matched by few. Now joined by our new companion, we make entry through the main entrance of the apartment complex. It smells of potpourri and mothballs. I don't know what it is, but older people have a thing for mothballs. Weird.

Clipboard in hand and my partner with the jump bag in hers we exit the bus. We grab the stretcher and have it in tow when we board the elevator and push the button for the second floor. I swear the elevator contractors need to pull their heads out of their asses when it comes to elevators. 2/3rd's of the elevators I enter were not built with the consideration of a stretcher in mind. They barely fit. At least the stretcher manufacturers have an I.Q.

and make the stretchers with the ability to collapse and or fold up.

The door of the elevator opens on the second floor of the apartment building. The three of us exit and make our way down the hall. The smell of the mothballs grows stronger and fills my nose with its chemical annoyance. We arrive at the apartment and knock on the door. I can hear a faint and muffled voice coming from within. He sounds in distress. Now my heart rate is up. The adrenaline pumping, the thump of my heart in my throat has me ready, prepared and able for whatever is behind this door. I know now that whoever is behind this door needs me. He needs help now. I get myself psyched up for the challenges that lie ahead of me. Cardiac, Diabetic, Respiratory and Neurological; I can work it. I am pumped!

Oddly enough the door wasn't locked. We make entry. We enter the apartment and are greeted by an odd aroma of urine, mothballs and a ripe adult diaper. There might possibly be a hint off mold on old dishes and rotting food smell present as well. Not too pleasant to my old nose, still we press on. The apartment is very small. My barracks room in the Navy was bigger than this shit hole. The cramped confines of this one bedroom nightmare are enough to make even a submariner claustrophobic. Clutter and random items are strewn about the apartment floor. Bags of old bed dressings, diapers and medical garbage fill the kitchen. If you are sitting there thinking this is disgusting, you are correct.

As we enter the bedroom, a feeble and decrepit old man lay before us. Withering away in atrophy. The resemblance between an Egyptian mummy and this man is uncanny. Covered in bedsores, unable to move let alone take care of himself my heart breaks. How can anyone just let another human being rot like this? "Sir, we are the Paramedics, did you need help?" "Yes" he says somewhat weakly. "Can you make me a cup of coffee?" "Excuse, me?" his query hits me with an astounding force. "Coffee, I would like a cup and the visiting nurse doesn't arrive until the morning." He acts as though this is status quo. My first reaction is that of anger. In a matter of milliseconds several responses enter my mind. "You pushed your medical alarm for THAT! GET YOUR OWN FUCKING COFFEE!" or possibly, "DO I LOOK LIKE A JUAN VALDEZ?" or even, "Only if I can have a cup too."

I finally decide on being professional and polite. "Sir that is not my job. If you are dying, have a medical complaint or need help, then and only then do you push that button. You can wait for your nurse to come in the morning. It is getting late, why don't you try and get some sleep?" His response is what I kind of expected and makes me wish that I had gone with one of my original three thoughts. "Well what fucking good are you? GET OUT OF MY HOUSE!" "GLADLY!" I snap back at him. My partner, the gentle soul that she is follows my lead and we exit. I half expected her to go make him the coffee and tuck him in for the night. She doesn't though. The officer walks toward the elevator shaking his head and chuckling. I don't blame him.

I grab the radio from my hip and press the key to talk. The conversation went like this:

251- "Dispatch Medic 251."

911-"Go ahead Medic 251"

251- "Yes Ma'am, we are going to be clear of the scene. There is no medical emergency here. The patient pushed his medical alarm button so we would make him a cup of coffee."

911- There is a pause. "I have no words. Show Medic 251 clear and available from the scene."

MYSTERY RADIO- The voice on the transmission is singing the old TV jingle, "the best part of waking up..."

251- I go with it, "... is Folgers in your cup!"

HEAT CASUALTY

USMC Officer Candidate School: Operation Bulldog
Quantico, Virginia 2000

I have been assigned to Bravo Company as the Company Corpsman and as the Platoon Corpsman for 4th Platoon. My job is to provide any and all emergency medical aid to the officer candidates for the Marine Corps as well as perform daily Med checks on the candidates. The Med checks consisted of fixing blisters, looking for trench foot and athletes foot. I would occasionally get candidates with a rash or fungal infection and if I was lucky a broken toe or two, possibly some sutures. It is the dead of summer and nothing can beat this Virginia humidity. The OCS is located right on the Potomac River and the humidity mixed with temperatures above 90 degrees makes the air is so thick you can cut it with a knife.

The staff at the Branch Medical clinic is top notch. The clinic has its own in house X-ray, Pharmacy, Lab even Physical Therapy. The back patio of the clinic is set up for rapid cool downs of heat casualties. Ice baths and 'kiddie pools' were set up so that a Marine on a litter can be sprawled across it and be rapidly cooled down in the event of heat stroke.

The clinic prided itself on the training and success rate of heat stroke treatments. We had dozens of Corpsman working through this clinic. Many like myself are assigned to the Platoons as field medical support. The rest work in the specialty sections of the clinic or run sick call. No matter where you were assigned, if a heat casualty came in to the clinic and you were in the building; your ass was out on the deck saving the Marines life.

One particular day the candidates were rucked up and marching on one of the back trails. It wasn't a huge march, only 5-10 miles or so. Right alongside them, I carried my medical pack which weighed at least fifty pounds. It would be more if carried enough IV equipment for the whole platoon. I was smart though and had already sized out each of the candidates for their specific IV size. I made each of the candidates carry their own IV equipment, so if one of them went down I just needed a bag of Saline and they already had the rest.

The march was uphill and on uneven terrain for a good while. The mosquito's bite any place they could get to skin. The trail is shaded but the cover from the canopy of trees didn't provide much in the way of relief from the heat. We push on through the suck and just embrace the fact that we're all in this together. We had been assigned a Humvee, which was at the rear of the formation. I could hear the droning of the engine in the distance. I would move toward the front of the formation and then back again. Looking for any sign of heat exhaustion or heat stroke. I occasionally find a Marine that has 'the look'. I simply tap them on the shoulder, "Drink water Devil Dog." They simply reply, "Aye aye Doc!"

We are about halfway done with the march when I hear the call. "CORPSMAN UP!" My Gunnery Sergeant is at the front of the formation calling out and waving for me to head up. I double-time it to the front. One of the candidates has collapsed. I drop to a knee and perform a rapid assessment. His skin is burning hot and bone dry. I take off my pack and call for a stretcher. "Gunny, help me strip him down." Gunny kneels down with me and we start stripping down the candidate. I reach into my pack and grab my thermometer.

"Pants too Gunny." Gunny looks up at me confused for a moment. I know what he is thinking, "I have to Gunny." He simply replies, "Pop him Doc." I insert the thermometer into his ass. It's the best way to get a body core temperature. The Marines dread this thing. They call it the 'Silver Bullet'. Funny, there is a beer with the same nickname and they both taste like shit. I get his temperature, 106 degrees Fahrenheit. I grab the Marines IV kit I had given him as I point to the radio operator, "Call the Clinic. Tell them I am coming in with a confirmed heat casualty. ETA 5 mikes!" The operator is on the horn, I start looking for an IV site. "Gunny, get these guys to drink water, we don't need any more going down."

"You Marines start drinking water right now! I want those canteens empty or Doc will pop a 'Silver Bullet' in your ass too!" I keep searching for an IV site as Gunny is pouring water from the downed Marines canteen on him. I can't find a site. His veins are retracted. No antecubital, no radial, not even a resident vein is visible. I have to do it. I spike the IV bag and move to the Marines head. I turn his head to the side and find my landmarks. "Really, in his neck Doc?" I just grunt at Gunny.

I insert my needle and get a good return of blood in the chamber of the needle. I set up my IV line and secure it. I start running Saline Bolus (wide open). The stretcher and the Humvee arrive. We move the Marine over to the stretcher and haul ass to the back of the Humvee. The Humvee tears off down the trail with the Marine and myself in the back. We are bouncing off of the sides of the Humvee and being tossed around like ragdolls as we race down the trail. I take out the few icepacks I have and place them behind his neck, in his armpits and in his groin.

The Humvee screeches to a halt and the back doors are flung open by several Corpsman, a Nurse and the Doctor who is a Commander. The team grabs the litter with the Marine and hurries over to the cool down pool. I am giving report to the Commander as the team works. A second IV is established in the patient with Lactated Ringers running. The Marine starts to become coherent somewhat as we scoop buckets of ice onto him. The shower above the Marine is dumping copious amounts of cold water on him as we fervently try to cool him down.

The Marine starts flailing around becoming increasingly combative. "Hold him down Corpsman!" The Commander shouts. I hold down the Marine's shoulders as another Corpsman is attempting to apply a non-rebreather oxygen mask. The more I hold him down the more he fights. The next thing I remember is seeing stars. The Marine candidate gave me a left hook directly in my jaw. The pain wasn't too bad however the chunk of my rear molar flying out along with a little bit of blood and hitting the nurse in her hair was enough to shock all of us.

"Are you alright Corpsman?" Now I am pissed. I know that the Marine's brain is baked and he has no control over his actions. I know this. Doesn't mean I don't want to return the favor. I rub my jaw, which is sore. I look at the Commander, "Yes Skipper. He just caught me off guard Sir." I wipe the blood from my lip as the group continues to try and cool down the Marine. "Go and see the Chief. Get yourself looked at, we will fix your Marine." I look at my Marine, "I'm good Sir. I'll stay, he's my Marine." The Commander looks a little pissed now, "Did I give the impression that it was an option Hospitalman Bowan?"

"No Sir. On the move Sir." I turn and walk into the building. The Chief Petty Officer gives me a once over and decides that I need to go to the dental unit on the main side of base. I go and get my tooth fixed. The fang fairies tease me about getting punched by an officer candidate. Whatever, Navy Dental Techs are just wannabe Corpsman. By the time I get back to the clinic the Marine had been stabilized and shipped off to the hospital.

Several days later the Marine had been discharged from the hospital. I had just finished my morning Med check with 4th platoon when he approached me. "Corpsman Bowan, I just want to apologize for my actions the other day..." I cut him off mid-sentence. "Listen Devil Dog. It wasn't your fault, your brain was fried and you are not responsible for your actions other than not hydrating correctly. This, you and me, we're good. Hoorah?" He looks at me gratefully and replies, "Hoorah Doc." I pack up my Med bag after having just fixed a gnarly blister on a candidate's foot. The Marine walks away stopping just short of the hatch by the stairs. He turns, "Thanks for saving my life Corpsman Bowan." I look up as I grab my cover. "Semper Fi brother."

THE CACKLER

Spring: Hospital Emergency Room

I am more than halfway through my Paramedic class and was precepting in the Emergency Room. It sucks that I have to go through school all over again but there is no reciprocity for Military Medics in the Civilian world. Basically the majority of people feel that Military Medics are less than Civilian Medics skills wise. Surprising thought that, seeing as how the Military develops most of the equipment and techniques these tools use now on a daily basis. Whatever, I embraced the suck and bit the bullet. Here I am, late at night sticking IV's into patients instead of being home with my wife and our newborn son.

The shift at the ER has been relatively boring. It is nothing like the STP (Shock Trauma Platoon) that I experienced in the service. I started a bunch of IV's and pushed several medications. EKG's and baseline vitals on most of the patients, all run of the mill type stuff. I had just done vitals and an IV on an elderly man about twenty minutes ago. His daughter brought him in because he "wasn't acting like himself..." very probably early onset of dementia.

I drew labs as per the ER doctor anyway. Maybe he has some chemistry that is off. His BSG (Blood Sugar Glucose) is normal, 137 so it is not a diabetic issue. His ammonia levels could be out of wack, he could have a nasty UTI (Urinary Tract Infection) maybe Sepsis; it could be a myriad of causes that can cause a patient to have altered mentation. The man seems harmless, frail in stature maybe 60 kilos (kilograms). He is about 93 years of age and you can see in his eyes that he is tired. Poor guy has lived a long life.

I was finishing paperwork with my supervising nurse when we hear a strange laugh. "He he he he" we both look at each other trying to figure out where that laugh was coming from. We hear it again, "He he he he".

I look at the nurse, "Did you just hear a cackle?" she nods yes. Out of the corner of my eye I catch a glimpse of wrinkly pink skin. "What the…" I must be seeing things. It's late and I have been here at the ER for over 12 hours. The nurse and I keep filling out my paperwork for class. A few minutes goes by and we hear it again, "He he he he…" the nurse looks at me and asks, "Where is that coming from?"

We soon get the answer when the poor old man from room 5 comes shuffling past us stark nude. I mean this crazy old coot had nothing more on him than what God had graced him with upon his birth. "Sir, sir you need to go back into your room…Sir." The nurse is now chasing after him as he continues to shuffle about and cackle. "He he he he" shuffle shuffle. "Sir, come back here." I can't help but watch this ER version of Keystone Capers with now two nurses and a naked old codger. Every turn the nurses make the old man counters differently avoiding capture. Cackling the whole time. "He he he he." He's pretty spry for a geriatric.

I honestly stood there and just watched. To this day it is hands down one of the funniest damn things I have ever seen. He reminded me of the children's story with the Gingerbread Man. "Run run as fast as you can you'll never catch me I'm the Gingerbread Man…" This goes on for a few moments until a Doctor returns to the ER and sees the events unfolding. "Aren't you going to help them?" the doctor asks. "I guess I should." I seriously have to control my laughter. "He he he he." Here he comes, he's like a slightly slower Road Runner going "Meep meep" and avoiding the Coyote. I step directly in his path and he stops.

He looks up at me with a shifty grin and a sly look in his eyes. "You're going to make me put my clothes back on aren't you?" I seriously am trying not to bust out laughing. "Yea old man, we need to get you dressed. You don't want to give these ladies a free show do you?" He smiles back at me as I gently escort him to his room. "Sure I do." I lose it and bust out laughing. "I was wondering when the big tattooed guy was going to help these dames." He is looking at me and for a moment it is almost like he knew what he was doing. Then he speaks to me, "You know Frank, I didn't think the Major was going to give us weekend liberty. Let's get off of this base and go get some dames and go drinking."

I have to compose myself. I now see that this poor man thinks I am someone else. The nurses put him back in bed and the doctor gives him 1mg (milligram) of Ativan to calm him down. Later talking to his wife, I asked her who Frank was. She said it was his best friend from the service. They were both with the 28th Infantry during World War II and that Frank had died at the Battle of the Bulge. My heart sank. I paid my respects and left for the night. As saddening as the story ended up, I could still hear his cackle the whole drive home. "He he he he."

EVIL

Spring

The shift had been pretty steady. Emergency calls and a few transports had occupied all of the crews that were on. The weather was warm with mild humidity. The air is filled with the smell of spring. My partner and I had just returned to the station a few minutes prior when the tones go over the radio dispatching the other two crews simultaneously for emergency calls. I look at my EMT, "I guess we're up again." He just nods and grunts. He never says a whole lot. He's a great EMT but he can be very taciturn. I start to log my trip sheets so I can knock out the paperwork. I had just sat down to start typing when the tones drop.

"EMS respond to Lakeview Drive for an unknown age male patient with the chief complaint of an abdominal wound. Police are on scene." Never fails. Every time I get a second to rest, oh well. My partner grabs the radio and responds. "County dispatch, Medic 4 acknowledges. Medic 4 enroute." We grab our gear and head to the truck. Light's go on and siren cranks up. Here we go again. We zip through the streets at a medium pace trying not to hit the people in the street.

God only knows why people around here feel the need to walk right in the middle of the street when there are perfectly good sidewalks on either side. The best part is when they finally move they give you a dirty look like you're in the wrong. We finally arrive on scene and tell the dispatcher such. I exit the truck and walk towards the Police who are standing next to a man a few feet away. There is also a middle aged gray haired woman standing next to the man. The patient appears to be in his forties. He is tall and slender, unshaven and unkempt. The pungent aroma of body odor is only equaled by the smell of sepsis emanating from his body. The patient is sitting on a brick wall rocking back and forth ever so slightly, mumbling and muttering. His hand held close in proximity to his mouth. He is barefoot as well. The moment I came into his peripheral vision his eyes locked on me.

The police officers are friends of mine and they begin to tell me some of the story. They were dispatched to a house a few doors down from our present location to arrest this guy. Apparently he was standing on a neighbor's porch and was exposing himself to the children at that location. They then proceed to tell me that they took one look at the guy and saw that he wasn't right in the head.

Now the lady with the gray hair speaks up. Her thick Russian accent almost impedes her English. She is very pleasant and appears genuinely concerned for the patient. I remember her now. She owns an assisted living facility that is just down the block. We don't go there very often as they have a contract with a private ambulance service for most of their ambulance needs. She proceeds to tell me that she had accepted this patient a few days ago and that he was not acting like this before. She also tells me that he wonders off for hours at a time and that some of the neighbors will bring him back to her facility. She then points out that he has a surgical incision in his abdomen that looks like hasn't healed correctly.

She lifts his shirt and shows me the gaping scar that appears infected and ecchymotic. The wound is approximately 5-6 inches in length. It stretches from his xyphoid process (bottom center of the rib cage) to his umbilicus (belly button). The whole time the man just fixates his eyes on me. Rocking back and forth slightly and still muttering. I try to interview the man but his glare is dark.

He never speaks although his lips move like he is narrating a book on tape. "Hey buddy, how are you feeling?" He doesn't respond.

"Do you want to tell me what is going on?" He just sits there, rocking and mumbling. I look into his eyes. There is nothing, no spark, no life. They're just empty. Usually you can look into a person's eyes and you can see 'them'. This guy, no such thing exists. His gaze pierces deep into my core. I turn to the Police and the Russian lady, "Well, he is obviously not behaving as a normal person should. Does he have any mental history?" the Russian tells me that he used to be in the State Asylum but has been bounced around between facilities since it was closed by the State.

Sadly, the Federal government cut funding from mental institutions and States followed suit. The last Insane Asylum in Pennsylvania closed its doors not too long ago and now these people are out and about. Sociopaths, Maniac's, Sex offenders, Pedophiles, Schizophrenics and the like are now among the general population of society because there is nowhere to put them. Yea politicians. Good job douchebag's. The Russian lady then tells me that she would like to have the patient evaluated at the hospital. This call is far from ALS (Advanced Life Support) but I can see that my EMT is uneasy with this guy.

Can't say that I blame him. The guy gives me the creeps too. I tell my EMT that I will take the transport. He is immediately relieved. The police tell me that they will follow us down to the ER and meet us at the door. I escort the patient to the truck picking up his shoes on the way. The man complies and walks with me never taking his black eyes off of me. I open the truck and seat the patient in the airway seat placing his seat belt around him. My partner hops in front and starts driving. I try to make small talk with the patient. He just sits and mumbles, and stares. "So, do you want to tell me what you were doing on that family's porch?" he laughs.

"A laugh, okay we're making progress. What were you doing on the porch buddy?" he goes back to mumbling. "I am just trying to help you friend, you want to tell me what you're thinking? How about why you were getting naked in front of some small children?" I really don't know why I asked that, but then he speaks up. "...if....if...the world were gentle...if it were gentle....I...I would eat the children's faces..." I sit back on the bench at this man's words. What the fuck did he just say? Every ounce of what is good in me wants to hit this fucker in the face. I don't.

I ask, "You want to eat the children's faces? What kind of sick shit is that dude?" he laughs and goes back to muttering never breaking his gaze on me. "That is some serious 'Hannibal Lecter' shit dude. Do you want some 'fava beans and a nice Chianti' too?" I don't know what else to do but then try to make a joke out of it, more for me than for him. Then he says something completely unexpected, "...I....I like you. You're funny...I will kill you last..." now I stand up. "Are we going to have a problem here buddy? I will knock you the fuck out!" in an instant his rocking and mumbling stops. His face becomes void of expression and those black eyes of his widen. "You will lose." Are the only other words he says to me.

We pull into the ER parking lot, the whole time the man just looks at me. I have my fist cocked and ready. I have seen things in my time, horrific and horrible. Military, Emergency Medicine, I was even a section 8 housing officer for a while, but nothing like this. This man may be septic, but I doubt that comments like that come from an infection. There are those that would argue with me on the matter, but they didn't look into those lifeless eyes. No remorse, no compassion and I swear no soul.

The back doors of the ambulance open and the police are standing there. The one officer who is a really good friend of mine sees my fist cocked back, "You all right brother?" he asks. "No dude, get this piece of shit out of my bus please." The patient willingly walks out of the ambulance always checking and looking for me. I am behind him, and he keeps looking back at me. We arrive at the Psych Nurse and place the patient in the 'Quiet room'. I give my report to the nurse and the attending physician. I make sure to warn them about this guy. I tell them everything and leave them with a warning, "Watch your ass with this guy. There is something not quite right with him."

My partner and I return to our bus and start heading back to base. I have never in all my time seen pure evil until I met this man. He still gives me nightmares.

SUNDAY IS JESUS DAY

Fall, night time:

We had been stead throughout the day as usual. The crews are hanging out in the crew room joking around and talking. My partner and I are the next crew up and we patiently wait for the next call to come in. Our patience pays off and we get dispatched top priority to the park down off of Chestnut Street for an unknown age female patient down on the ground. Possible cardiac arrest." We run to the truck and mount up. The garage door opens and the lights come on. My partner calls enroute to the dispatcher and us race out with sirens blaring. The roads are wet and slick. We proceed cautiously. I can see emergency lights in the side mirror. One of the other Medic trucks is backing us up.

The dispatcher comes over the radio, "Units responding to Chestnut Street, police are on scene stating that the patient is breathing." We acknowledge the dispatcher and continue on. We arrive on scene to find several police cars already on scene. The officers are standing around a park bench with their flashlights focused on the woman that is lying there. I exit the truck and start walking over while I put on my exam gloves. "Howdy boys! What do we have here?"

My brothers in blue look over and they each are wearing a smile on their faces. "Hey Spike, look who it is!" Oh, God. It can't be that serious if they are talking like that. They part like the Red Sea and there she is. In EMS you tend to get 'frequent fliers' and Virginia here is one of the finest. This woman stands at least 6 feet 4 inches. I swear that she could be a linebacker for the Steelers if she weren't smoking crack cocaine and drinking a gallon of cheap vodka every day. Her eyes are open and she is talking to the police. I have to shake my head. Several times a month we take

Virginia here to the ER so she can detox and then she gets released and she does it all over again.

"Virginia darling! Hey sweetie, what did you do now?" she looks up at me and smiles. She likes me. I am one of her favorite Medics. I should be, I see her enough. I brought her out of overdose last year and ever since I have been her 'tattooed angel'. She sits up and looks at me, "Oh Spike. I think I over did it again?" I can smell the booze from ten feet away. "No Virginia, I have seen you over do it before, this seems to be one of your better days. You want to go to the ER?" she nods a yes and staggers to her feet. The rubber neckers start to come out as we walk toward the truck.

One of the onlookers is this weird but nice guy that always rides around the city on his bicycle. He isn't all there in the head but he is harmless and always saying "God Bless you brother." And "Jesus loves you!" he's cool. As I walk Virginia to the bus I ask, "How much crack did you smoke today Virginia?" she dodges the question at first and then finally responds "A whole bunch." I shake my head, "Sweetie, do you smoke crack every day?" she promptly responds as the bible bicycle guy is walking his bike past my truck. "I smoke crack everyday but Sunday. No crack on Sunday, that's Jesus day!" "Amen sister! No crack on Jesus day!"

I turn and look and bible bicycle guy is wheeling away singing at the top of his lungs, "No crack on Jesus day, hallelujah!" I look back at the police and my partner who are now pissing their pants laughing. I escort Virginia into the ambulance and we take her to the hospital.

THE JOCK STRAP

Camp Pendleton 2001
USMC

I had just finished a day of sick call and training. The usual barracks antics ensued. Some of the Marines are playing volleyball, some are cooking out on the grills near the smoke deck. Different types of music fill the air, everything from Hip-Hop to Heavy Metal. I was making my way back to my room when I hear one of the Marines calling out to me. "Doc! Doc! You got a sec Doc?" I turn and see one of the guys from my Platoon coming towards me. "Yea, Martinez, what's up?" Martinez is kind of hobbling toward me. I was thinking that maybe he hurt himself doing PT (Physical Training) or something.

He frantically hurry's toward me as fast as his body will allow. "Doc, umm...can you take a look at something for me?" I now notice that Martinez is holding his groin. Damn it, he got an STD (Sexually Transmitted Disease) I start to think. I take out my keys and unlock my room. I swing the door open and let the cool air blast us in the face. I left it on all day because I knew that the temperature was going to be scolding hot today. "Welcome to my off duty clinic." I say as I usher him in.

Now by no means to I carry the equipment or medicine to diagnose and treat a STD in my barracks room. I can at least take a look and see what's going on before I have him come to sick call in the morning. If it is a STD the poor Devil Dog is going to have to get his 'bore punched'. A 'Bore punch' is Corpsman slang for swabbing his urethra. We stole it from the rifle range where the instructor takes a rod and rams it down the barrel of your rifle hitting the bolt slamming it forward to ensure the weapon is clear. Are we getting the picture?

I close the door and turn around seeing that my Marine already has his trousers and boxers down. How he got naked that quickly is beyond me. Before my eyes is the biggest, most swollen, red and infected penis I have ever seen. This thing is infected to the tenth degree. I know male horses that would be jealous of what this guy was packing. "Umm… Damn Martinez! Is…umm…are you normally that big?" he looks up scared as hell and says, "No Doc. I mean I'm a decent sized dude but this thing is fucking huge and it hurts! I can barely walk Doc!"

I can see that there is some sort of crust alongside his thighs. I grab my med bag and take out a pair of exam gloves. "When did this start Martinez?" I was just barely touching him and he writhes in pain and growls at me. "Arrggh… Damn Doc! Don't fucking touch it!" I snap him a quick look, "Martinez, you been sleeping around with some skanks or trophy hunters?" Trophy hunters are women that hang around bars and clubs looking for single servicemen so they can marry their dumb asses and get a free ride. Housing, Commissary, Medical care etc… Much to their surprise when they find out that a majority of Enlisted Military families have to go on Welfare because the government doesn't pay us dick.

Anyway, he quickly replies "No Doc! I haven't been sleeping around and I know I didn't get it from my girlfriend because she broke up with me a few weeks ago and this just started last week." Maybe it's not a STD. "You said this just started last week? So what, you woke up one morning and were ready to start making porno's?" he gets a little chuckle. "No Doc. I woke up and I had a rash down there. So I put some cream on it. The next day it got bigger and started to hurt. Over the next few days it kept getting worse so I put more and more cream on it."

"Son of a bitch!" I declare allowed. He looks scared at my comment and possibly a little relieved that maybe I know what this is. "Martinez, did you use hydrocortisone?" he nods yes. That's it. Fungal rashes react violently to steroids like hydrocortisone. They spread like wildfire. The steroid is like 'miracle grow' to the fungus. I explain all of this and then tell him to come to sick call in the morning. "Doc, isn't there something you can do now?" I shake my head no, "Short of calling an ambulance for you to go the base ER not really. If you want I will be happy to drive you over to the Naval Hospital on base and get you seen."

He quickly dismisses the notion and says that he will embrace the suck until the morning. I tell him to maybe ice it down every so often to help reduce the swelling and also to take some Motrin. Ahh, Motrin, a Corpsman's best friend. We prescribe Motrin like its candy. The running joke in the service is that Motrin is all we carry in our bags. This is not true I have acetaminophen too. Joking. So Martinez leaves with a little bit of Motrin that I give him and I close my door. I take off my gloves and go to the head (bathroom) to wash my hands.

I have a few beers and ready my uniform for the morning. The next day we go to PT and then shower and chow. I put on my camies and head over to sick call. There is Martinez sitting painfully and anxiously. The poor guy damn near fell out of his chair as I walked in. "Easy Martinez. Let me go talk to Chief and we will get you fixed. Alright?" He nods a painful yes. I go into the back and talk to the Chief Petty Officer who is the IDC (Independent Duty Corpsman: Exact same training as a physician's assistant only not a commissioned officer) and I tell him what is going on with Martinez. He agrees with my assessment and has me confirm it with a Woods lamp. (Most fungus will glow green underneath a black light)

I bring Martinez back to the exam room. He drops his drawers and Chief comes in to see for himself. "God Damn!" Chief calls out at the sight of Martinez' member. I have to try not to laugh. Chief turns out the light and I turn on the lamp. Holy shit, it looks like Martinez' junk walked through a vat of nuclear waste it glowed so damn much! We turn on the lights and Chief tells him to use the cream that I will get him and to use several jock straps to keep his manhood supported. Ice it down, Motrin etc... Martinez leaves and that is that.

Or so I thought. A few days later, we had a Battalion run. Every company in the Battalion is there. Half way through the run here comes the Master Gunnery Sergeant and Martinez running back from the front of the column. Master Guns yanks me out of line. "Doc, this hard charging Marine here says that you can explain to me why he has to wear so many God Damn Jock Straps that his crotch looks like a cod piece in my Battalion formation! Is this true Doc!" I look down at Martinez' crotch. "What the fuck Martinez? How many did you put on?" The Master Guns is getting pissed, he looks at Martinez "Well? Answer your Corpsman Marine!"

Martinez is turning red from embarrassment. "Umm...like 7 Doc!" I snap back "7? Are you kidding me?" The Master Guns is no longer pissed, just confused as hell. "Well yea, Doc. That's how many it took to fit it all in." I turn to explain everything to the Master Guns. He cuts me off before I can even get a word out. "Doc! I don't want to know! I really don't want to fucking know! This is obviously some medical thing that you are treating and squaring my Marine away, so let's just leave it be!" he snaps at the both of us, "Is that understood?" "Aye aye Master Guns!" we both reply. "Good! Now get the fuck back in formation Doc! You too Corporal Jock Strap!"

From that day on, Martinez was known as Corporal Jock Strap.

THE JUNKY THAT WASN'T A JUNKY
(But actually was a junky)

(But she swears she isn't)

(But she is)

Winter: Nighttime

Running EMS in an urban area that has a respectable crime rate is always an adventure. There is always something going on and you always get to see some of the most brilliant examples of humanity. (I'm being sarcastic) Don't get me wrong, there are decent human beings here. It's just that the majority of them are piss ass scared to come out of their homes at night. Hell sometimes even in the day. It is what it is. We had just received a call for an unknown age unconscious female, possible cardiac arrest.

My partner and I exit the truck at the address and are looking for any sign of anybody. The house is on a back cut alley that parallels a hillside. There are no visible lights on in the residence and nobody is answering our voices. I know that a second Medic unit is on its way to back us up and the Police are just arriving on scene. We ask dispatch to do a call back and they do. The caller says to come in through the front and come down the stairs. The police enter first with their weapons drawn. We have no clue what is inside waiting for us so I don't blame them.

The outside of the house looks like a shit hole. The paint is chipping off, the gutters are hanging down from the roof and there is garbage scattered throughout the yard. The inside of this residence however is immaculate. Floral print wallpaper, tea cozies and gold rim tea sets are on the dining room table. The place reeks of potpourri and looks like a little old lady lives here. "Police! Anybody here?" The officer calls out. We hear a scuffle in the basement. "Hello Police and Medics!" the officer calls out again. A voice answers back, "Uh...yea. Uh...down here. She's down here."

We all head down the cumbersome stairs. The officer first with his sidearm drawn. Then I go with the jump bag and the monitor. My partner and now the second Medic crew follow after. The basement does not even remotely resemble the upstairs. It is dirty and grimy. The cement floor has garbage everywhere along with dirty clothes. It smells like mildew and trash. Underneath the stairs the guy that lives here built a room. It is tiny, maybe 5 feet long by 3-4 feet wide. Inside is a tiny single bed with an old TV and VCR next to it. There is also a nightstand that has syringes and empty stamp bags (1 gram of Heroin is called a stamp bag because the bag it comes in is the size of a stamp) on top. There is even a spoon to cook up the shot with.

The female patient is in her mid-twenties and is a known prostitute in the area. In fact one of my first calls with this company was bringing this chick out of over dose. I noticed that the guy that called 911 was her 'John' (customer) and that he was trying to fasten his zipper on his jeans. I look at the patient and see that her pants are undone as well. "You sick fuck! She OD's and you finish the transaction before we get here? What the fuck is wrong with you?" The police now see what I see. They scoop up the 'John' and start hauling him off. I look at the patient. She has agonal respirations of 4. She is pale and unresponsive. I grab the prefilled syringe of Naloxone out of the jump bag and jam the needle into her thigh.

The Naloxone will stimulate her respiratory system and also block the cell receptor sites to prevent the opiate from working. 2mg in the leg should get her going while I look for an IV site. She doesn't have many options. There is a ton of scar tissue at most of her veins, plus fresh tract marks. This is a big reason I hate IV drug user overdoses. The other medic with me suggested using an IO drill (Intra Osseous drill: drills right into the bone marrow giving access to admin drugs and fluids). "Not yet brother, she has a good EJ (External Jugular) right here. I don't want to have to drill her if I don't have to.

I prep the site and start my line. With the needle in her neck, this is when the medicine starts to work and she wakes up screaming! "God damn it hold her!" My partner and the other crew pile on top of her trying to hold her as she screams and kicks and flails. "What are you doing to me? Who the fuck are you fucking fuckers?" You can see that she was burdened with an overabundance of schooling. "We're the Medics and we're trying to save your life!" I have my knee on her shoulder now as my left hand tries to keep her head down and my right hand tries to maintain control of the needle that is in her Jugular vein.

"What? Why? What is happening?" she screams at everyone even the police. "You overdosed and damn near died! Now hold still!" she is confused and frantic. "What do you mean that I overdosed? Why can't I get up? Let me up mother fuckers!" the other crew is holding her legs down as she kicks. My partner is holding her arms and I have her upper torso and the needle. "Stop moving junkie! I have a needle in your neck!" she just becomes more and more pissed off! "Why is there a needle in my neck? GET IT OUT!" The line blew. It would have been a good IV if she had held still. I remove the needle and control the bleeding with sterile 4x4 gauze.

We release her and let her move freely. "What do you mean I overdosed? I'm not a fucking junky asshole!" before I can even respond Josh the EMT from the other crew chimes in, "Yea right! Shut up junky!" she looks around rapidly. "I am not a junky! I have never done drugs before in my life!" She must still be high, we have all taken her to the ER for overdose before, and every police officer in this city has busted her for prostitution at least once. "Shut up and hold still before you bleed out." She gets flustered like a three-year-old crossing her arms and pouting.

We start to escort her to the ambulance. "I ain't going to no fucking hospital!" I look at her, "You don't have a choice." She quips back, "the hell I do? I don't have to go if I don't want to. Plus you fuckers keep calling me a junky! I ain't no fucking junky!" I have to pretty much push her toward the ambulance. "Sure you are. You're also a hooker. You don't think I know you but I do." She rips her arm away, "No you don't asshole! You don't know shit!" I laugh in her face, "Sure I do. I brought you out of overdose during one of my first shifts here in the city. I also know that you have Hepatitis C and that your 'pimp' I mean 'boyfriend' is going to be pissed when he finds out you OD'd again."

"Oh, my God! You're right. He is going to be so pissed off at me!" I smirk at her, "See. I know you. You knew that I knew you were a junky right?" she shrugs my comment off. We finish escorting her to the truck and are able to calm her down a little. We get her to the ER and were able to establish a tiny 24 gauge IV in her thumb. It's all she has left. I gave her some fluids and some more Naloxone along with some oxygen. We transfer her to the nurses in the ER where she tries to deny again that she is a junky. "Shut up junky!" the nurses say, they all know her too.

I have all the respect for a person that wants and tries to get clean. I will support a recovering addict or alcoholic 110%. But if you don't want the help, don't want to quit and blame everyone else for your screw ups and then deny you have a problem while the needle you used is sitting next to you; then I have no respect for you. If you want help, I will help. If you don't want help and you want to end up damn near a corpse that you're 'John' still has sex with while you die, fine. I will call the coroner when we find your corpse in an alley.

TICKLE TEST

Springtime.

God I hate paperwork! I'm not even halfway through the shift and I can't get any paperwork done because these jokers won't get off of Facebook. "Hey are you guys doing trip sheets or what?" I wish there was some sort of work ethic around here. Finally he's done on the computer. "Thank you." Now I can get some paperwork done and then grab something to eat.

Of course. I sit down to get my paperwork done and the emergency tones drop. "Station 250 please respond, 1314 Opal Way, for a 17 year old female with chest pain and shortness of breath. Family states that the patient is in and out of consciousness." I pile up my trip sheets and place them in my mailbox as my partner grabs the radio. "Dispatch, station 250 acknowledges the call on Opal. Medic 251 will be responding." We grab our coats and head for the truck room.

"Received Medic 251 responding at 1811 hours." My EMT Mike climbs in the driver's seat and starts the truck. I open the garage door and hop in the passenger's seat. "This is such a bullshit call! Isn't this that girl we always go to? You know the one that 'passes out' or 'seizes' every time her and her mother get into an argument?" Mike is probably right. Statistically 17 year old girls don't get chest pain. Unless they have a congenital heart problem or something severe like that. This girl however is a full on drama queen. I fell for her act the first time and gave her the five star treatment, when she faked a seizure. I know she was faking because I was trying to call command to get orders for Valium. I couldn't remember how old she was at that time so I asked my partner. She stopped mid seizure and answered "17!" then proceeded to seize again. I can't wait to see what this dumb ass has in store for me this time. "Dispatch Medic 251 is enroute." Mike turns on the lights and hits the siren.

Opal Way isn't that far from the station, we should get there rather quickly. Mike is driving like an idiot as usual. I have to hold on to the 'Oh Shit bar' on the door to the point that my knuckles are white. "Hey man, where do you want to eat after this?" I am starving. "I don't know dude, how about Mexican food?"

Holy Shit that guy just ran a red light and almost side swiped us! "You mother fucker!! You didn't hear the damn siren or see the flashing lights? You cocksucker!" Mike has a real way with words. "Yeah, Mexican sounds cool. I could definitely chow down on a burrito or two."

We arrive on scene to find that the police are also on scene. Apparently they had been called for a domestic dispute at the same address. "Dispatch Medic 251 is on scene with police." Dispatch acknowledges that we're on scene and we exit the rig. I grab the jump bag and make my way inside. The patient's mother is standing at the top of the stairs screaming like always. "What the fuck took you guys so long? My daughter is lying in there dying and you're just walking!" I can see where the patient gets her knack for the dramatic.

We enter the bedroom and the 17 year old patient is lying on the bed 'passed out'. I kick the bed, "Come on Chrissy! Get up!" she doesn't move. Her mother becomes even more upset. "How dare you! My daughter is sick and you come into my house behaving like that! I'll have your badge for this! She has epilepsy!" I turn to the mother, "Really? What epilepsy medication is she on then?" the mother stops and thinks. "Ummm...I don't know..." Of course she doesn't know. That's because the patient isn't on any.

"You mean to tell me you're her mother and you don't know if your daughter takes medication for her epilepsy?" I look at the officer who asked the mother the question and I try not to laugh.

I knuckle rub the patients sternum, "Come on Chrissy! We know you're faking it! Knock it off!" She doesn't budge. I lightly flick her eye lashes with my finger, "Chrissy, Chrissy, wake up." Still she doesn't move. Her mother chimes in, "You see asshole? I told you she is genuinely sick!" I shoot a glance back at the mother. I still have an ace up my sleeve. "Is she now?" I reach down and tickle the patient under her arm pit, "Coochey coochey coo!" The patient bursts out laughing and then glares at me evilly. "You're an asshole!" she says. The mother now becomes irate. "You were faking it! You little tramp! What the hell is wrong with you?"

The officer looks at me and says, "Only you dude!" We leave so that the Mom and the daughter can resume their fight while the police stay to mediate. "Dispatch Medic 251, we're clear with no medical emergency."

NO LEG TO STAND ON

Summer:

It was a hot July day and my partner and I had been running are asses off doing transports and emergent calls all shift. We were heading back to the station when the dispatcher from the 911 center drops are tones. "Station 230 respond, E3 (low priority) to the corner of Main and 4th street for a 48 year old female with leg pain." Sounds like a bullshit call and of course we are the only crew available. "Dispatch, Medic 238 acknowledge and enroute." The call is only a few blocks from the station. We make our way down the road with no lights and sirens.

As we arrive on scene we see a scrawny woman standing on the side of the road with a leg cast on her left leg. "Her leg is broken, no wonder she has pain. These people get dumber every day." My partner isn't wrong there. I grab the radio and call out on scene with dispatch. The woman seems and acts like she is high. She smiles a rotting toothed smile at me as she fumbles and tries to hide her crack pipe in her pocket.

"Ma'am, did you call the ambulance?" she manages to get her pipe put away and then answers my query. "Yea, yea I did. My leg hurts and I need some morphine." Typical med seekers. First words out of their mouths when you arrive on scene is for morphine or fentanyl. "How long has your leg been broken?" she looks down at her leg and then back at me. "Are you going to give me pain meds or not asshole?"

Her pungent aroma hits my nose and turns my stomach. I then notice her eyes. Aside from being under the influence of narcotics I notice something else. The sclera (white portion) of her eyes are jaundiced. She either has cirrhosis of the liver or she might even be septic. Her hands tremble and writhe back and forth over one another. "How long has your leg been broken ma'am?" she looks back down at the filthy cast. I can see that she is trying not to put weight on it and any amount of pressure causes her pain.

"It's been broken for a year, now can I please have some medicine?" A year? Holy shit! "Ma'am, when were you supposed to have the cast removed?" she is becoming more and more agitated. "Just give me the medicine!"

She nearly collapses onto the pavement as I catch her mid fall. My partner rushes to the truck and retrieves the stretcher. We place her on the stretcher as she is fading in and out of consciousness. I check her carotid and radial arteries for a pulse. It's faint. "Let's get her in the truck. I'll get her I.V. and place her on the monitor. Get her on some oxygen and let's see if she has any I.D." My partner nods and we get into the truck. As we lift the stretcher into the back of the ambulance the smell of her cast is rancid and becomes increasingly worse.

I begin placing the leads for the monitor and as I attempt to place the left leg lead I notice a black and green purulent fluid oozing out of the cast. "What the hell is that?" there are maggots floating in it. That's just nasty! I place her on the monitor and see that she is in sinus bradycardia. Her heart rate is about 42 beats per minute, her respirations are 8 time a minute and her blood pressure is 82/36. I start an IV in her jugular vein as that there are no veins left in her arms or legs. Habitual IV drug users are often like this.

I administer an IV bolus of 250cc's normal saline and raise her legs to prevent her from going into any further shock and keep what is left of her blood volume towards the trunk of her body. My partner starts driving the bus to the hospital with lights and sirens blaring. I administer a dose of Naloxone although it might not work. I check her blood sugar, 419. Her heart rate is picking up a little and the smell of her leg and the ooze is getting worse. I notify the hospital of my patient and we soon arrive.

The doctor meets us in the exam room along with several nurses. I give my report and then tell the physician that the patient had stated that she has had the cast on for a year. His eyes widen and he orders a nurse to retrieve a cast saw. He examines the cast and as he pushes on it the ooze squirts out of the top. The cast is pliable. "That's not normal, right Doc?" he shakes his head. The doctor cuts off the cast and cracks it open like a coconut. The stench is so immense that two of the nurses began vomiting immediately.

Maggots pour out of what is left of her leg. The necrotic flesh is clinging to the cast along with what is left of her muscle tissue. The decay and maggots have eaten her leg down to the bone. My stomach turns upside down. I have seen some horrific things in my time but this is one of the top 5. The patient was shipped up to surgery quickly where she had her leg amputated. The patient then spent several weeks in Intensive Care to be treated for sepsis and blood poisoning.

THAT DOESN'T HAPPEN IN EMS! (Quick and short stories)

-While transporting a patient to the trauma center I witnessed another Paramedic crew WALK a patient with a slit throat into the emergency room while the patient held his own pressure on the wound and carried his own bag of IV fluid. No reprimand befell that Paramedic crew.

- I witnessed an ER doctor fly a patient from his ER to a trauma center. This is not normally a problem except the patient had Do Not Resuscitate papers, Bi-lateral Hemopneumothoraxes, a AAA (Abdominal Aortic Aneurysm), end stage cancer, end stage renal failure, was on hospice and that had been resuscitated multiple times. The MD had disregarded the patient's valid paperwork stating that they did not want life saving measures and never contacted family to see what their wishes were. The MD then cost the family an approximate $14,000 transport bill for the helicopter and he then quipped, "...glad I'm not getting that bill..."

-Patient had been shot in the head and his brain matter littered the passenger seat of the vehicle he was sitting in. The attending Paramedic (not me), decided to work the patient and transport him to the nearest hospital. The patient's brain matter was riding shotgun mind you and the patients eyeball was about to fall out of his head. The EMS crew transports, performing CPR and arrives at the ER. After a few minutes the ER staff was able to get a faint pulse back with a dropping blood pressure. Not entirely unbelievable, the patient's brainstem is intact along with the medulla oblongata; it is feasible that some vital signs could return for a brief amount of time. The attending ER MD decides to fly the patient out. As the EMS crew is transferring the patient along with the medical evac crew, one of the EMS crew members looks at the patients bulging eye and says, "You eyeballing me boy?"

- I had just returned to the station after a long and grueling day. My partner from my other shift I work was returning to the base at the same time. She steps out of the truck in tears. Her weeping only briefly interrupted by her attempts to gain control of her breath. I quickly rush to her side and ask what is wrong. She proceeds to tell me the following story. That they were dispatched to a residence for a 14 month old female with a possible rectal bleed. Upon her examination of the child she discovered that there was blood coming from the little girl's rectum and vagina, but also semen. The 14 month old girl was raped by a family member in the household. No media coverage was done.

-When I was a young EMT just a hair past 16 years of age I had the misfortune of responding to a female patient versus a freight train. The train obviously won, and we remained on scene to aid the medical examiner retrieve the pieces of the woman that had committed suicide. While we were picking up her body parts, the medical examiner picked up the woman's head and asks, "Anyone want some head?"

- I was partnered with a real piece of shit for a Paramedic. We'll call him Schmuck. The guy was so pretentious and yet so lazy that I was stuck by two different used needles that he had left out in a one week period and he had the balls to say that "...he would never do anything like that..." and that it "...sucks to be me..." One day we were working a cardiac arrest and he was attempting to intubate the patient when the patient vomited directly into this Paramedic's mouth. I couldn't help but laugh my ass off while performing compressions. Once he stopped puking himself I couldn't help but ay this. "Hey dude, you know what the most interesting thing is about other peoples vomit?" He looks up at me as his skin is turning green. "It tastes just like your own." He throws up again. Karma bitch!

SHE WAS FINE A MINUTE AGO

We were dispatched to a "skilled nursing facility" for an elderly female patient that was having a change in mental status. My partner and I arrive to find the patient lying in bed with her eyes closed. The "nurse" had stated that the patient wasn't responding to the staff and that she "just wasn't herself". I reach down to gently shake the patient and see if she is awake. The patient doesn't respond and she is cold to the touch. I check her radial and carotid pulses finding none. I then notice the base of her arm and see that morbid lividity has already set in. I look to my partner, "Dude! She's been dead for hours!"

This shit pisses me off. I walk out into the hallway and down the hall to the nurses' station where the charge nurse is gabbing on her cell phone. "Excuse me, Ma'am?" she shoots daggers at me with her eyes. "I'm going to have to call you back, the ambulance driver needs something." She hangs up her phone, "Yea? What?" the attitude aside I have little tolerance for incompetence. "Yes Ma'am, Hi. Can you tell me how long the patient has been dead?"

The nurse becomes immediately defensive and dismissive, "What do you mean dead? She's not dead! I just got a blood pressure on her!" I crack up laughing right in the nurse's face. "Oh, really? What was this pressure?" The nurse is not amused by my laughter, "120/80! I don't appreciate you laughing either!" This excuse never ceases to amaze me. Whenever a healthcare provider slacks at their job and doesn't want to take a blood pressure they use the 'text book' answer of 120/80.

Her bullshit excuse only makes me laugh harder, "Really? 120/80? How do you get a blood pressure on a patient that has been dead for over six hours at least?" The nurse stands up shoving her chair backward and she storms off down the hall cursing at me. "Fucking ambulance driver! You don't know how to do your damn job! She's fine, let me show you!"

The nurse actually goes into the room and proceeds to shake the patient's corpse. "Wake up!" Okay, I have had enough. I reach for my radio, "County dispatch Medic unit 237." The dispatcher comes across the radio, "Dispatch, I need a Code Zero time and a County Police unit to this facility for a DOA." The nurse turns to me quickly with eyes wide and scared. "Medic 237, that's received. Your Code Zero time is 1421 County Police have been notified."

The nurse begins fumbling through her words, "Police? Why are you calling the cops?" I proceed to fill out the 'Dead on Arrival' paperwork for the coroner as I answer her question. "Well Ma'am, when a patient dies in a county run facility and the ambulance driver, we call ourselves Paramedics by the way, suspects suspicious circumstances; the coroner and county police are called in to investigate."

"What mother fucking suspicious circumstances? She was fine a minute ago! I got a blood pressure!" I decide to promptly educate the 'nice' nurse. "Ma'am that is physically impossible. Let me educate you about lividity. Lividity is when in a time frame of approximately 6 – 12 hours the blood vessels begin to break down in a deceased body. The blood pools to the lowest parts of the body because of gravity. In this patients case this would be the bases of her arms, legs, and back. It is usually dark purple in color as we can see here on the patient, but what do I know? I'm just a dumb ambulance driver and you're the nurse that got a blood pressure of 120/80 on a dead body."

She walked away.

SELF INDUCED VASECTOMY

I had just recently been let off of provisional command as a Paramedic and was now a full-fledged Paramedic. I was sitting in the dispatch office of the station signing for my narcotics box when we heard a gunshot down the street. Not uncommon in this neighborhood so not much was thought of it.

I walk down into the truck room and begin checking my truck along with my partner. A few moments goes by and a man comes up to the garage door. "Hey you guys, my buddy has been shot around the corner!" I pull my eyes from the paperwork on my clipboard. "What? Where is he?" the man points down the street as he runs off. I grab my radio and call it in. We wait for the police to show up on scene to ensure that the area is secure.

They give the all clear and we proceed in. The house was actually at the end of the back alley behind our station. We exit the truck to see a man lying on his front porch writhing back and forth in blood soaked sweat pants. "Where are you hit bud?" I grab a trauma dressing with my gloved hands. The man is screaming in pain, "Oh God!"

My partner starts cutting off his pants. "Sir, where are you hit?" he grabs my arm and squeezes as he answers. "My balls! I'm shot in the balls man!" My eyes must have widened something fierce. We expose the wound and sure enough, three wounds. In through the right nut, out through the left nut and into his thigh.

His leg is bleeding profusely and I notice that I can see the bullet just under the skin. I direct my partner to apply pressure to his thigh. My boss had walked down the alley to assist. He's a damn good Medic from Ireland and his medical skills are exemplary. He has retrieved the stretcher from my bus. The police are asking the victim who had shot him. "I don't know man! Some dude! Some dude I don't even know walked up and shot me!"

I look at the wounds and start to think for a moment. "Sir, you mean to tell me that some dude walked up and placed the barrel of his gun perpendicular to your scrotum and shot you through both of your balls?" We move the man to the stretcher as he answers, "Yea man! That's what I'm fucking saying!"

I may not be a police detective, but I am a military veteran. I have seen many things in my life and the facts just aren't adding up here. No shooter in the history of the world would walk up, wielding a gun and be able to get their intended target to hold still enough to 'place' that shot. It's easier to just kill the target. One of two things is happening here. Either the shooter had a very personal grudge against this man's testicles or the more likely scenario is that Mr. Homie 'G' Thug wannabe here went to put his illegal pistol into his sweat pants and he shot himself.

In the back of the ambulance I start an IV and run some normal saline to replace lost fluids. His heart rate is fast but normal on the monitor and his blood pressure is stable. "Give me some fucking meds man!" The guy is screaming like a child. "Answer me a question here bud. Who really shot you?" He opens his eyes and looks me in the face, "I already told the pigs! Some dude!"

I speak before I think, "You know if the cops ever caught 'some dude' the world would be a much safer place. Think about it; who robbed that bank? 'Some dude.' Who killed that guy? 'Some dude.' Who sold those drugs? 'Some dude.' Some dude is the biggest criminal offender on Earth."

The patient doesn't look to happy with my rant. "You mean to tell me sir that 'some dude' walked up to you with a gun and placed it against your scrotum and pulled the trigger?" He nods, "Yea man! That's what I'm saying! Now give me some fucking pain meds!"

I start dialing the hospital to get a hold of a doctor for the authorization to administer the pain meds. "You know sir, I really think you're lying and the truth is that you went to put your gun in your sweat pants and accidentally pulled the trigger shooting yourself through your boys. I'm right aren't I?" The patient turns his head and mumbles a yes. I get approval for 50 micrograms of Fentanyl with a secondary dose of 50mcg if need arises. I administer the meds and we begin transport to the trauma center. The trip is uneventful minus a question from the patient. "I'm gonna lose my balls aren't I?" I'm not going to lie to the guy, "Probably dude."

When we arrive we are hurried into the trauma bay. The doctor asks for a report. "42 year old male patient with chief complaint of a self-inflicted gunshot wound to the scrotum. Negative loss of consciousness, conscious alert and oriented times 4; PERRL (pupil's equal round reactive to light) negative JVD (jugular vein distention) Trachea is midline; No shortness of breath or chest pain, lung sounds are clear in all quadrants bilaterally; Abdomen soft and non-tender in all quads bilat. There are three penetrating traumas that resemble gunshot wounds in his pelvic area here. It looks like the round entered through his right testicle, passed through the left testicle and into his thigh. I have two large bore 14 gauge IV's in his arms with normal saline running and I have administered 50 mcg of fentanyl IV push."

"Anything else?" The doc asks. "No Doc, just the self-inflicted vasectomy."

HICCUP

So I walk in to the ER with my partner and a patient on the stretcher. It is almost midnight and the shift looks like it is going to be an 'all-nighter'. One of the other Medic crews was also entering into the ER with their patient. They had been dispatched for a male patient with a rectal bleed. As they walk through the ER, their patient is screaming and cursing like a sailor.

I look at the Medic from that crew who is a longtime friend and ask what's wrong with the guy. "Dude, I'll tell you later." The expression on his face is that of shock and disbelief. My partner and I drop off our patient and I give a report to the nurse. No sooner than I finish my care report we receive a call for an overdose patient.

We quickly clear up and head to the overdose. We pick up and treat the patient heading back to the ER. I drop off this patient and give report to the nurse who is not thrilled to see me again. The Medic from the other crew runs up behind me and grabs my arm pulling me aside. In his hand is a print out of an X-ray.

"So apparently, my patient and his wife were having some happy naked time. The guy can only 'get off' with rectal stimulation..." A myriad of objects come into mind as to what this guy shoved up his ass. The Medic holds out the X-ray to show me. I can only say, "...but how?"

The X-ray showed a flashlight. Not just any flashlight, this is one of the gigantic 'D cell Mag-Lights' The kind that takes four D-cell batteries. The damn thing is ALL THE WAY UP! Even the beveled edge! My jaw must be on the floor. The attending ER physician walks up behind us.

"Hey guys what's going...is that the guys X-ray from room 2?" The other Medic and I say nothing. We just nod our heads in unison. The Doc is flabbergasted, "How did he get the bulb section in there? What did he do? Hiccup?"

BLIZZARD

In 2010 the Pittsburgh area was hit with a nasty blizzard. Nobody was ready for it. The snow fell so fast that most places couldn't get their plow trucks out of the garages let alone on the road plowing and salting the roads. We were trying to deal with the plethora of calls that came pouring in with no 4 wheel drive trucks.

The call comes in for a 15month old baby boy, unresponsive. Not breathing. My partner and I go as backup for the Medic crew who was next up. The call is two towns over and what should have been a three to four minute drive in normal weather conditions becomes a ten to fifteen minute ETA. Our trucks couldn't even get up the hill across the street from the base.

Hands freezing, wind blasting our faces with snow; we get out of our truck to help push the Medic truck in front of us up the hill. We even used branches from a nearby tree to put under the wheels to try and give it some traction. We finally get their truck rolling and we use the same trick to get ours up the hill.

Lights flashing and reflecting off of the snow as it falls, it looked like something from Tim Burton's nightmare. Cars sliding all over the road and smashing into parked cars, even our own trucks were fish tailing and sliding so badly that if we went over 15 miles per hour we were going to wreck and die. There were no snow tires on the trucks and the company we worked for is way too cheap to buy chains for the trucks.

We are almost on scene when the County dispatcher informs us that the Police are on scene and CPR is in progress. "Oh God!" I hate pediatric calls, always have. Now we know this little boy is seriously in bad condition. We arrive on scene behind the other ambulance. I can see my buddy Dave hop out from the truck and sprint into the house.

I tell my partner to help the other Medic set up and I follow Dave into the house. I reach the first landing of the steps and I see one of the Policemen doing compressions and cheek puffs on the child as he passes the child to Dave. Dave resumes compressions and makes his way to me.

He passes the child off to me and I start compressions on the little boy and I am running for the truck as I give rescue breaths. I enter the truck and place the child on the stretcher. The Medic tells Dave to just go and asks me to stay with him. The door slams shut and I continue compressions.

The Medic grabs the pediatric defibrillator pads and places them on the child. The truck starts moving. "Asystole! Keep doing compressions." I continue the chest compressions, feeling the boy's sponge like rib cage accept the force of my hands with no resistance. The Medic grabs an I.O. needle and drill. (Intra Osseous: into the bone)

He cleans and preps the site on the boy's leg and drills the needle into the boy's bone marrow. Good, now we have a line. "Pushing Epi!" The Medic administers the Epinephrine 1:10,000. "No shock, keep up compressions!" I do as he asks. The truck is sliding back and forth on the road. This makes it even harder to work in the back especially with the wet floor.

The Medic places an ET tube (Endo Tracheal) and checks his placement by listening to the boy's lungs and abdomen to make sure that he has a patent airway. The tube is good and the Medic secures it. I continue my compressions as we head down the road.

I look at the little boy as we work. Thoughts of my own son pop into my head.

My son is the same age. I focus and continue working. The Medic passes the BVM to me. (Bag Valve Mask) Now I am bagging the child and doing compressions at the same time. The Medic keeps checking the monitor and administering the cardiac meds. We have no idea how long the child was down and we are heading to the closest trauma center. We have been trying everything.

The Medic even did a manual defibrillation. Normally you don't shock asystole, but I understood why he did it. He wanted to give this kid every chance possible. I would have done the same.

The truck swerves violently sending my head slamming into the cabinet next to me. Apparently PENNDOT (Pennsylvania Department of Transportation) has two salt trucks on the road that spun out and almost hit our ambulance. Thanks to Dave's driving we survived and evaded certain death. After 45 minutes we arrive at the hospital. The trip with lights and sirens in normal weather conditions is about 8-10 minutes.

We rush into the ER where the medical team waits for us. The Medic gives the report along with everything we did. My eyes never leave the sight of the little boy. We have been working on this kid for almost an hour. The ER team works him for three minutes when the doctor asks if anyone has any objection to calling time of death. No one answers. The doctor makes eye contact with me and he can see that I want them to keep going.

The look he gives me back is that of a mentor to a pupil. His eyes tell me that there is nothing else we can do. "Time of Death: 2215."

CHUCK NORRIS

It's been one of those days. Running my ass off, call after call they just keep coming. I finally get a moment to smoke a cigarette and drink some coffee when we get a call to assist another Medic truck from another township. They have a male patient that was ejected from a moving vehicle.

I leave my cup of coffee sitting on the wall next to the ER and rush to the truck. My partner starts up the old war pig and flips the lights on. "County dispatch, Medic 268 is on the way." We zoom through the streets and drive up the ramp leading to the road where the accident happened.

I exit the truck and see the Medic from the other service is a friend and relatively new Medic. He's a good kid, he's just a huge spaz. I see the patient lying on the ground his legs spread out like a frog. This isn't going to be good. I already know the guy has an "open book pelvic fracture" and that we are going to need a helicopter.

"Spike, oh thank God! Help me here man!" I walk up and start assessing the patient. "What do you have Matt?" Matt looks at the patient and starts telling me what he has done and found as he is splinting a compound fracture of the patients arm. "The patient here was a passenger in his girlfriend's car. They were arguing and he didn't want to be party to her yelling anymore. So genius here jumped out of her car as she was making the bend there at approximately 45-50 miles per hour."

I have had some seriously nasty fights with my wife in the past, but nothing so bad that I would jump out of a moving vehicle. "So, Spike...um do you think we should fly him?" It's his patient, I'm just here to help. I can see in his eyes that he is piss scared. I am going to have to do this, damn it. "Yes Matt. Call the bird. It's rush hour and by the time we stabilize this pelvis and get him in the truck it can already be at the LZ."

The patient is in and out of consciousness. I grab a sheet off of the stretcher and roll it up. I slide it under his buttocks and tie and cross over making a diaper splint.

Its old school, but it works. Used to be that we could use M.A.S. Trousers (Military Anti-Shock) but the damn ER's kept cutting them off of the patients. Damn things cost about $2000 a pop. I check for pedal pulses and find that they are very faint. We get the patient immobilized and into the ambulance. An EMT puts the patient on high flow oxygen as Matt and I establish large bore IVs.

We are going to have to replace a ton of fluid. The guy's abdomen and thighs are swelling up with blood from his pelvic fracture. The patient opens his eyes. "What is going on?" I talk and keep working on the guy. "You're in the back of an ambulance buddy. We are working on fixing you." The patient becomes a little violent, trying to fight his way off of the backboard. I pin his head down with my forearm, "Where do you think you're going?"

He swats at my arm, "Let me go mother fucker! I'm fine!" I press harder on his forehead with my forearm. "Oh, sure. You're the poster child for fine. Arm fractured, internal bleeding and a pelvic fracture that may end up killing you. You're all manner of fine." He shoots me a dirty glance. We arrive at the LZ and the flight crew comes into the back of Matt's bus.

"Hey Spike, sup Matt. What do we have here?" Matt and I both know the flight crew fairly well. "Well Steve, the action star here didn't want to continue his fight with his girl so he jumped out of her car at around 50 mph." Steve chuckles a bit, "must have been some fight?" We continue the report and transfer care over to the flight crew who has kept the helicopter hot and running.

The patient looks up at me just before we leave his side, "Why? Why did this have to happen to me?" I blurt out a response before I can even think, "Because you jumped out of a moving car thinking you were Chuck Norris. You're no Chuck Norris dude."

THE TUNNEL

In part of the service area that we cover there is an old tunnel leading to a scarcely traveled back road. This tunnel is rife with ghost stories. Legend says that there is a ghost of a green man that walks the tunnels at night killing any who see him.

I love a good ghost story as much as the next person, but this was a different kind of gruesome death. My partner and I are called to the tunnel for a report of a man slumped over his steering wheel. We arrive to find that man has been shot in the head and has long since shuffled off this mortal coil.

Gun still in hand it looks like a suicide. We call the police and they come down with their investigators and what not. Something is bugging my though. The glass on the window is blown into the compartment. There is a small wound on the dead guys left temple and a huge open cavity on the right side of his head. The gun is in the man's right hand. A 1911 45 caliber pistol. That's a huge caliber round.

I point out my concern to the police chief and to another police officer. They promptly tell me that it's a suicide and that I should mind my own business. "The sheer physics of this situation says that it's a homicide and someone staged it to look like a suicide. The gun is in his right hand. The exit wound is on the right side. The glass of the driver's window is blown in."

I am quickly dismissed and told to return in service. No wonder there is such a high unsolved homicide rate in this town. I walk back to the truck and my partner tells me to calm down. "Dude, you're not a cop." I acknowledge him and we start to drive away. I am just aggravated. A trained monkey could look at the scene and see that it was staged.

Over the period of a few weeks after this call, I kept getting calls to the tunnel. Some during the day, some at night. The last time I got a call there it was for an overdose lying in the middle of the tunnel. My partner and I were down on the ground working with poor lighting. I sent my partner to get the stretcher from the truck.

I hear a shuffle off to my side and I glance over to see a green wisp of smoke waft away into the darkness of the tunnel. Chills run down my spine and the hair on the back of my neck stands straight up. I grab my flashlight and search the area quickly for any sign of what I had just seen.

My partner returns and asks what I am doing. "You didn't see that?" I tell my partner what happened and he laughs me off. We get the patient loaded on the stretcher and lift the stretcher up when I realize the spot we are in was the exact same spot of the fake suicide guy. I look back to where the green smoke was and I catch a glint of metal on the ground. I shine my light down and there it is.

A spent 45 caliber bullet. Lying on the ground, right where the green smoke was. I grab an extra exam glove and pick it up wrapping it inside. We wheel the patient to the truck when I realize that the round was in the trajectory of a bullet that would have been fired through a window, through a man's head and out the other door. If he had shot himself, the round would have exited left through the window spewing glass and brain matter out the driver's door and onto the wall of the tunnel.

We treat our patient and drop them off at the hospital. I then have my partner head to the police station where I inform the desk sergeant of my findings and I turn over the bullet. A few months later an arrest was made in the murder of the man from the tunnel. I never would have found that bullet if it weren't for the green smoke.

Be sure to check out and read my other works:

War in the Backyard

War in the Backyard: Region 3

Coming Soon:

The Comic Book Apostle

War in the Backyard: The 4 Judges

Long Road to Georgia

Check out our Facebook page:

www.facebook.com/spikebowanauthor

www.facebook.com/irregularmischiefproductions